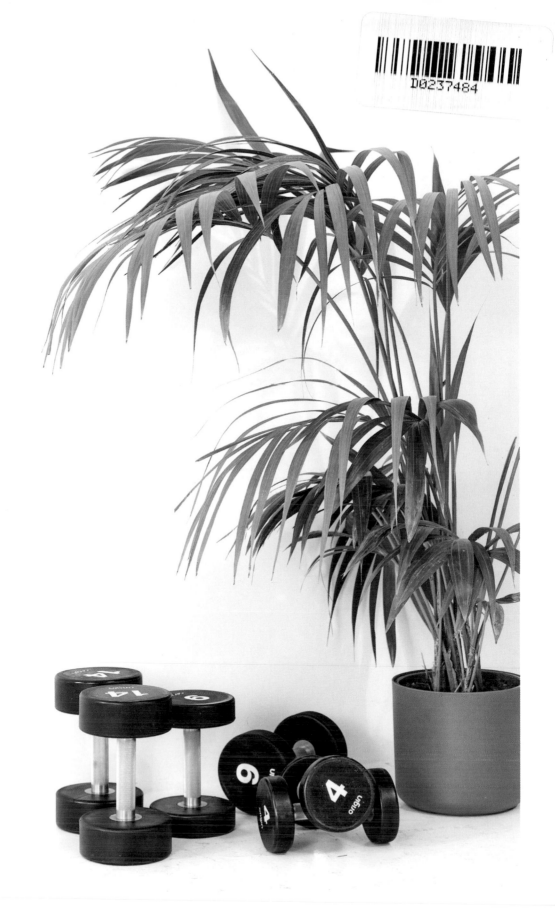

This book is for you, the reader.
May you never have to go on a diet again!

101 WAYS TO LOSE WEIGHT

AND NEVER FIND IT AGAIN

SCOTT BAPTIE MSc

Photography by Jack Lawson

Hardie Grant

QUADRILLE

CONTENTS

Welcome to the only weight-loss book
   you'll ever need 7
How we lose weight 8
How to use this book 9

Nutrition & eating habits

 Exercise & fitness habits

 Mindset & motivation

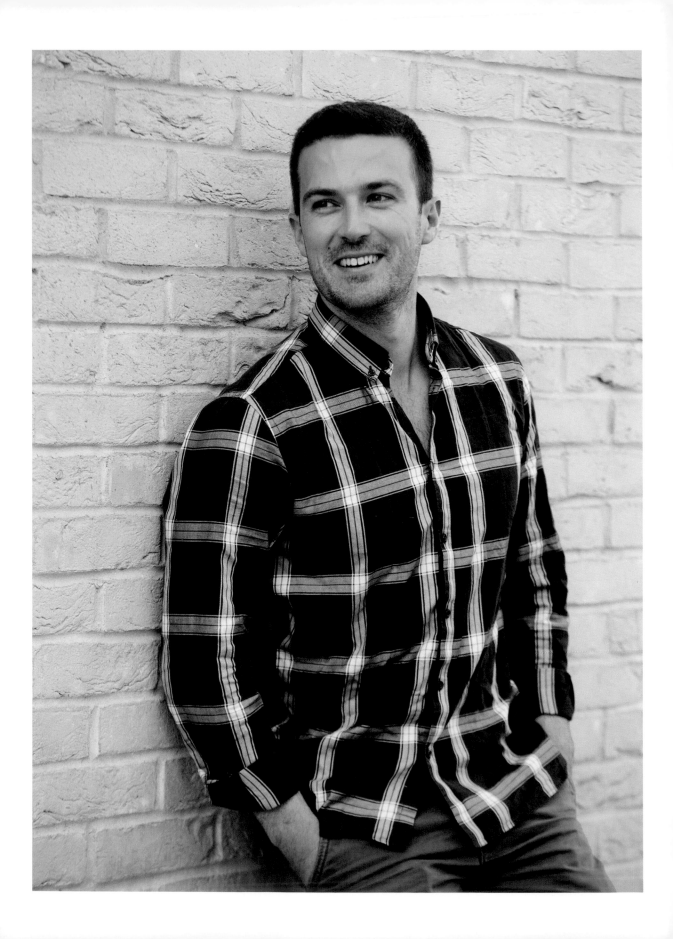

WELCOME TO THE ONLY WEIGHT-LOSS BOOK YOU'LL EVER NEED

I've got some good news for you. If you're fed up with diets, 'clean eating', relentless fitness programmes and depriving yourself of your favourite treats, you've come to the right place. Your days of vegetable juice and superfood powders are over. You'll never need to take another fat-burner again, you won't have to re-mortgage to buy the latest detox kit, nor will you have to force yourself to eat only brown rice because that's what the magazine said...

I'm going to be the encouraging voice in your head, the parrot on your shoulder, your weight-loss coach in your pocket, and together we're going to fight the fat so that this will be the last weight-loss book you'll ever read.

Once you've finished with this book, not only will you feel motivated, inspired and lighter, but also...

- You'll discover that individual foods are not to blame for weight gain and most nutrition advice is based on myths, hearsay, anecdotes and pseudoscience.

- You'll be able to recognise and avoid unhealthy 'detoxing', 'cleansing', 'rebooting' or any other popular, unsustainable fad diets and will not be fooled by their empty promises.

- You're going to learn 101 ways to lose weight, supported by scientific evidence, covering nutrition, exercise, sleep, goal-setting, mindset, food environment and willpower that will help you to get leaner, fitter, stronger and happier without the hunger and heartache.

But before we go any further, it's important to understand the basic mechanisms behind how we lose weight.

HOW WE LOSE WEIGHT

There are two words that, when combined, create the foundation for weight loss: calorie deficit. If a calorie deficit doesn't exist, YOU WON'T LOSE FAT. Quite simply, a calorie deficit is when you consume fewer calories than you're burning – or you're burning more calories than you eat and drink per day. When this happens, your body starts to look somewhere else for fuel. Body fat is loaded with energy, so when you're in a calorie deficit, your body turns to fat for a fuel source. Body fat is burned and, ta-da! you lose fat, and weight, as a result.

» **If you've ever lost weight, it's because you've been in a calorie deficit.**

» **If your weight isn't going down, it's because you're burning roughly the same number of calories as you're eating.**

If your weight is increasing, it means you're in a calorie surplus – that's when you're consuming more calories than you're burning.

Most of the unpleasant diets you might have tried in the past have the same core tenet: they create a huge calorie deficit that involves you eating next to nothing or exercising for hours upon hours every day. Sure, you might lose a lot of fat in the beginning, but the diets are often so horrible and unsustainable that you only follow them for a few days and, in most cases, the weight just goes on again when you've finished.

But that's not going to happen this time.

HOW TO USE THIS BOOK

You're not going to do anything so extreme or unpleasant that you feel that you want to throw in the towel and go back to 'normal' after a few days.

This book is full of ways and habits that you're going to practise – not rules that you follow – and that you'll get better the more you do them. Most of them are going to help you to create a small calorie deficit (because that's more sustainable than anything drastic) by either reducing the calories you eat or by increasing the calories you burn.

But don't panic. Calories count, but you don't have to count calories.

Anyone who tells you that calories don't count should be ignored; you can't argue with physics. However, most of the habits we're going to cover will move you into a calorie deficit without your having to weigh every gram and write down every morsel of food you eat. Yes, there are some habits that do focus on tracking and will require some logging on your part, but you don't have to pick those ones to follow if they're not for you – they're just another tool that you might pick from the 101 tools in this box.

My suggestion is that you start off with 3 ways to adopt for the next 30 days. Pick the ones that you think are the most realistic, the ones you'll easily be able to follow, the ones that sound the most fun and the most enjoyable. Each month you'll tack some new ways onto the ones that are already in place. So, after 30 days you'll add on another 3 ways to the ones you've already been practising, after another 30 days add on another 3, and so on.

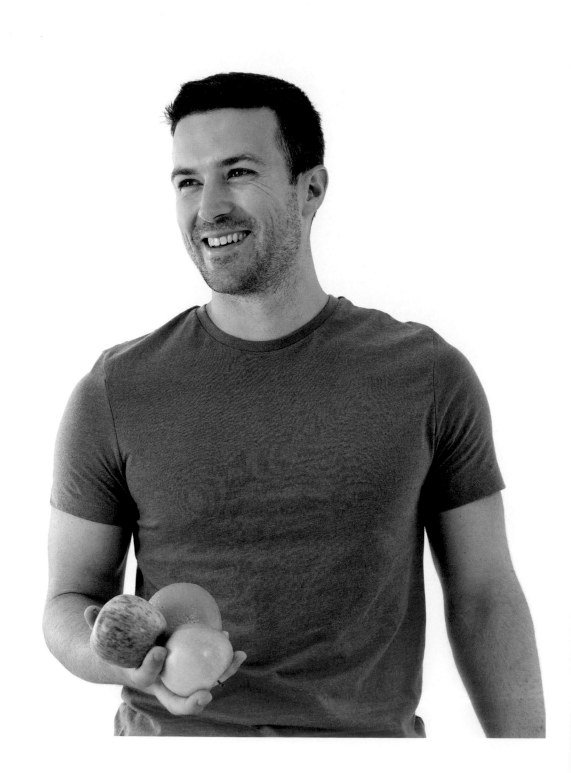

Why only 3? We're setting the barrier low. My mate Karl uses a quote that I love: 'It's better to be consistently good, not occasionally perfect'. There is nothing stopping you from trying to implement 10, 20 or even 30 ways all at once, but it would involve such a huge change to your current lifestyle, you'd be likely to forget a lot of what you're applying. Also, because it's so different from what you do 'normally', it won't be much fun.

Biting off more than you can chew, pun intended, often results in people becoming 'work-week dieters'. As diets always start on Monday, they find that they are so 'good' during the week that, come the weekend, their extreme restriction and bird-food diet causes a blowout and wipes out the calorie deficit created during the week. Sound familiar?

If you pick small habits to focus on every day, you will develop a level of consistency throughout the whole week, instead of your week being a mixture of extremes: perfect Monday to Friday, the weekend a disaster, only to repeat the cycle the following Monday. Consistency of effort is greater than intensity of effort, and it's that consistency that will produce stunning results over time.

Before you get started, check out the hidden resources that accompany this book. I've created a really helpful habit-tracking diary that you can download for free here: weightlossbook.co.uk/resources

Bear in mind that this is not a fitness manual, so I don't explain how to do every exercise I talk about. I want to help you develop tricks for manageable and long-lasting weight loss by showing you ways of approaching exercise and fitness (and nutrition, of course). So if you need guidance on how to use a kettlebell, or what a burpee is, check out the resources page mentioned above.

1. DITCH THE DIET MENTALITY

Diets are like boats: you go on them, you come off them. They're like books: you start, you finish, you go and do something else.

Diets just don't work.

If they did, and I'm guessing you've tried a few, you wouldn't be reading this book. It's been reported that 48% of people in the UK have tried to lose weight in the last year[1] and almost two thirds of that group said they do so 'all or most of the time'. Unfortunately, national statistics show that many are unsuccessful. Despite the prevalence of dieting, obesity in the UK has tripled in the last 30 years, with 24% of British men now obese (second highest rate in the world) and 26% of British women obese (also the second highest rate in the world).[2]

So, what's the problem? Diets are generally characterised by a rigid set of rules that ban 'forbidden' foods that are supposedly making you fat: no carbs, no sugar, no meat, no dairy, no fruits, no fat, no fun. They encourage you to eat a load of things that you don't like: who's for a spinach, kale and buckwheat smoothie? They're short term, often promise rapid results (6lb in 6 days, anyone?), force you to reorganise your life and are often based on pseudoscientific nonsense. All in all, they're generally pretty unpleasant.

One of the biggest flaws with dieting is that restriction increases food cravings; studies have shown this time and time again.[3] If your diet bans bread, you want more bread. If you go on a chocolate detox for 30 days, all you can think about is chocolate. The biggest problem is that once the restriction has been lifted, you're more likely to eat to excess compared with if you hadn't placed the restriction upon yourself in the first place.

'... rigid eating behaviors lead to food cravings thereby hampering long-term weight maintenance. Indeed, people with flexible control strategies have been found to be more successful in long-term weight maintenance.'[4]

» Here's an idea

Why make healthy eating harder than it needs to be? Your biggest restriction should be to avoid unnecessary restriction.

So, before you go any further in this book, make a promise to yourself that your days of dieting are done and dusted.

You're not going to make a tonne of dramatic changes all at once; you're going to make small, simple changes that accumulate over time. You're not going to ban any foods, anything can be enjoyed in moderation. You're not going to try and lose 6lb in 6 days, you're going to focus on the process, not the outcome. You're going to do things differently!

TAKE-HOME HABIT

Diets suck; habits rock!

2. WALK OFF THE WEIGHT WITH A STEP TRACKER

Walking has to be one of the most underrated ways to ramp up your calorie expenditure. When folk think of exercise they imagine noisy gyms, sweaty bodies and high heartrates. If that doesn't do it for you, it's cool, go for a walk instead.

It's low impact, it's free, its super-accessible, it's sociable and it's really effective for helping you lose weight.[5]

Thanks to the popularity of wearables like a Fitbit® or the Apple Watch®, walking has almost become a competitive sport. It seems like everyone is on a quest to hit their daily 10,000 steps. In 2017, more than 310M activity trackers were sold which generated over $30 billion![6]

There are several reasons why these step-trackers are so great. Firstly, they ramp up your calorie expenditure. If you're going to be on your feet and walking more then it's a no-brainer that you're going to burn more calories as a result.

Wearables also keep you accountable as you can set activity reminders to go and do 250 steps every hour, or if you've been sitting down for too long they can also give you metaphorical nudge to get moving.

Most of the trackers also have a community element that lets you compete in challenges with your friends who have similar devices. You could do a daily or weekly step competition, see who can climb the most flights of stairs in a day, and so on.

Setting a quantifiable step-goal is also a low barrier to entry when it comes to setting exercise targets. If you do zero exercise, saying that you'll start going to the gym 3 times a week is unlikely to be realistic. A step target is much easier. Park the car further from work, only take the stairs, get off a bus or tube stop earlier and walk the rest of the way, only take the car if the destination is further than a mile away. The easy, realistic and attainable habits that will boost your step count are endless.

'I probably do 10,000 steps a day anyway.'
Actually, you probably don't.

When it comes to estimating our steps or energy expenditure (the calories we burn in exercise) we're terrible. Folk generally overestimate the calories they burn in exercise by 3–4 folds.[7] That's another reason why a step-tracker is better than just estimating how much, or how little, you actually move.

TAKE-HOME HABIT

Get yourself a step-tracker and commit to a daily target like 5,000 or 10,000 steps per day.

3. CURE CRAVINGS WITH DIET DRINKS

Hold on a minute… Surely a nutritionist can't be recommending diet drinks; don't you know they're full of chemicals?

If there's one topic that is guaranteed to get knickers in a twist, agitate the gym bunnies and get you unfollowed on social media, it's diet drinks.

Why something as insignificant as a can of soft drink generates such an emotional response and is the cause of so many heated debates is, quite frankly, bizarre.

Listen to some people and they'll have you running to the hills in fear. You may have heard that diet drinks cause cancer, that they trick your body and turn on fat-storing mode, they deplete nutrients, make you hungry… The list goes on.

Most of the 'facts' surrounding diet drinks are simply a load of nonsense. For starters, there is no evidence[8] that sweeteners cause cancer in humans, and they certainly don't cause weight gain either. In fact, the complete opposite has been shown: switching from a full-sugar drink to a diet drink can help you lose weight![9]

Ever craved something sweet? Of course you have. Sometimes artificially sweetened foods, although unlikely to serve any nutritional benefit, can eliminate sugar cravings. If a zero-calorie diet drink is the drink of choice instead of its 300-calorie, full-sugar counterpart, then that simple switch could make a big difference to your waistline.

Let's say you have a 500ml bottle of fizzy drink with your lunch every day and you switch to the diet version. Just like that you've reduced your calorie intake by around 2,000 per week, and you can do it knowing that the evidence shows that it's safe to do so.

Now, some studies have shown that people who are overweight or obese drink more sugar-free drinks than people who are a healthy weight.[10]

But is the diet juice to blame? Unlikely.

These studies have shown that the overweight people – who were drinking the diet drinks – also had a much higher calorie intake than those who didn't. What's more, people who generally have poor diets may be more likely to drink diet drinks to offset the number of calories consumed by making poor, high-calorie food choices.

Although overweight people may drink more diet drinks, the diet drinks are unlikely to be the cause of the problem. This is a classic example of why correlation does not equal causation. Here's another example: in America, in summer, people eat more ice cream. In America, in summer, more people also get eaten by sharks. One does not cause the other. Ice cream does not cause shark attacks nor do shark attacks cause ice cream sales to flourish, just like diet drinks don't cause obesity.

TAKE-HOME HABIT

Swap any full-sugar fizzy drinks that you consume for the diet version, or go for a no added sugar juice, water or fruit tea instead.

4. AVOID THE 'SEE-FOOD DIET'

We love the see-food diet. If we see it, we eat it.
We're all the same, especially when it comes to Easter time or Christmas: when we're swimming in selection boxes or chocolate eggs our willpower is tested by all the sweet temptations.

An easy tip to conserve your willpower for when you really need it is to make unhealthy eating a hassle.

The old adage 'out of sight, out of mind' comes into its element when you're trying to lose weight. If you keep junk food on the kitchen table top, you'll eat more. Put it in the cupboard and you'll eat less; put it at the back of a low cupboard behind the blender you never use, and you'll eat even less; store it in the garage and you'll probably forget it's even there.

Studies have shown this to be an effective tactic. One alarming bit of research found that if people kept a box of cereal on their kitchen counter they were around 20lb heavier compared with people who kept the cornflakes in the cupboard. If they kept fizzy juice in plain sight, they were around 25lb heavier compared with people who didn't.[11]

Although this study only had around 200 participants and was based in one town in New York, so may, therefore, not be representative of what goes on in households elsewhere in the world, it still suggests that we're all prone to the see-food diet.

Some other things that you can do to make unhealthy eating a bit more inconvenient is to avoid bulk buying calorie-laden snacks and sweeties from the supermarket; buy only what you need there and then and don't keep big tubs of ice cream in the freezer.

If you've got kids in the family who like a sweet treat on occasion, that's fine, but try not to keep a stash in the house. Instead, take a walk or a bike ride to the shop or go out for an ice cream. You'll make it more of an occasion, you'll be able to have some quality family time, you're less likely to overeat and, if you walk to the shops you'll boost your step count and burn some calories in the process.

TAKE-HOME HABIT

If you've got some tempting foods that may sabotage your progress in the house, make sure they're kept out of sight. If it's more inconvenient to get to them, you're less likely to eat them.

5. PILE ON THE PROTEIN AT BREAKFAST

Protein is a way to win at breakfast!

Not only does it help repair your body after exercise, but more calories are required to digest protein than fat and carbohydrates (this is called dietary induced thermogenesis). Research has shown[12] that people who eat protein at breakfast have better appetite control and reduced hunger throughout the day.

For most folk, breakfast is a way to feel full, top up essential vitamins and minerals, minimise mid-morning hunger and give you a mental boost too. Having a meal first thing is also especially beneficial for people working out before lunchtime or performing a manual labour job.

Some high-protein breakfast ideas that you can try include yoghurt (go for the natural or Greek variety instead of the fruit kind, which is often sweetened), eggs, smoked salmon or some lean meats like ham or turkey on toast instead of jam or marmalade.

Here's a great recipe for protein pancakes:

1 scoop whey protein powder
100ml [7 tbsp] milk
1 large egg
50g [½ cup] porridge oats (blitzed in a blender to a fine flour)
1 tsp ground cinnamon
¼ tsp baking powder
light cooking spray, for the pan

Put all the ingredients in a bowl and beat well to combine and form a batter. Heat a lightly oiled frying pan over a medium-high heat. Pour some of mixture into the pan then tilt it in a circular motion so that the batter coats the surface evenly. Cook the pancake for about 2 minutes until the bottom is light brown. Loosen with a flexible spatula or fish-slice, flip over and cook the other side for half a minute before serving.

» **Here's an idea**
Adding a scoop of protein powder to your morning porridge could also be a simple way to get a protein fix at breakfast.

What about a smoothie?

This is one of my favourites that I have to kick-start my day before I head to the gym. Just whack all of the following into a blender:

50g [½ cup] porridge oats
1 scoop whey protein powder
250ml [1 cup] water
50g [½ cup] frozen blueberries
pinch of ground cinnamon

Foods to avoid in the morning would be highly refined, low-fibre, sugar-laden carbohydrates (sorry Frosties® and Crunchy Nut® Cornflakes) as they don't really fill you up, they're not good for your teeth and can cause an energy slump mid-morning. Instead, opt for high-fibre carbohydrates to complement your protein, like wholegrain oats, muesli, fruit or multigrain bread.

See also Power up Your Protein with a Shake on page 58.

TAKE-HOME HABIT

Make a habit of including a source of quality protein with breakfast each morning. I'm sorry to say that whilst it may be protein rich, a fat-laden full English breakfast doesn't count!

6. HOP ON THE HIIT BANDWAGON

High Intensity Interval Training (or HIIT for short) isn't a new style of training, but thanks to the likes of Joe Wicks and other Instagrammers, it has been given a new lease of life.

With short, snappy and intense workouts that need no equipment, it's easy to see why so many are ditching their steady-state cardio in favour of a HIIT workout.

Here are some of the reasons why.

» It's a time saver

One of the standout highlights of HIIT workouts has to be the fact that most workouts are over and done within 15–20 minutes. This can be great if the thought of a 45–60-minute steady-state cardio session, like a run, is your idea of hell on earth! Typically, most HIIT workouts will start with a warmup. This is followed by 15–30 seconds of high-intensity exercise (let's say burpees for an example), followed by 30–60 seconds of rest. You'd then repeat this for several rounds and you're done before you know it.

» HIIT is extremely versatile

You can do hundreds of body weight workouts in your own living room, in the park, in a hotel room, etc. No gym membership required and they're extremely versatile. Get a stopwatch or timer and some empty space and you're good. Due to the popularity of HIIT, a quick YouTube search will return hundreds of results so you won't struggle with a lack of variety.

» It's great for heart health

One meta-analysis[13] (a study of other studies) found that it significantly increases cardiorespiratory fitness by almost double that steady state cardio in patients with lifestyle-induced chronic diseases.

(cont.)

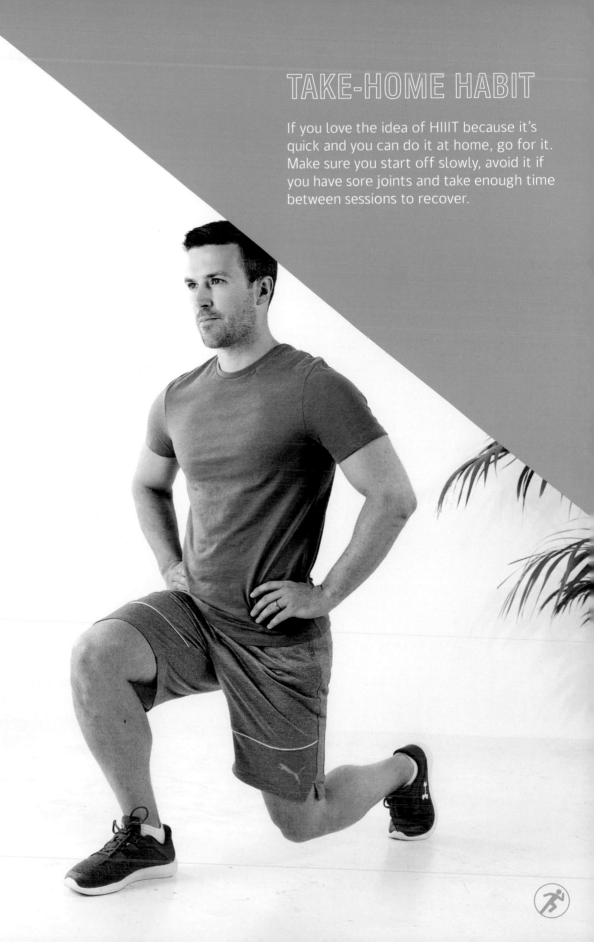

TAKE-HOME HABIT

If you love the idea of HIIIT because it's quick and you can do it at home, go for it. Make sure you start off slowly, avoid it if you have sore joints and take enough time between sessions to recover.

HOP ON THE HIIT BANDWAGON

» It's proven to burn fat

There are a lot of published studies that show it can help burn fat. A study in the *International Journal of Obesity*[14] found that doing HIIT 3 x per week reduced total body fat and increased insulin sensitivity.

» HIIT can suppress your appetite

The good news is that a recent study[15] found that you can suppress your appetite with only 2 minutes of HIIT! As little as 4 × 30 seconds of 'flat-out' cycling was sufficient to suppress appetite and reduce a the hunger-inducing hormone, ghrelin.

Before you go and ditch your traditional run around the park or a cycle to work, it's important to know that a recent meta-analysis[16] comparing steady-state cardio with HIIT found there were no significant differences in fat burning when the two groups were matched for time or energy expenditure.

This means that although HIIT is a good fat-burning tool, you can still stick to your morning run or cycle if you prefer. HIIT is just another tool in your arsenal.

7. GO WITH THE GRAIN & EAT BREAD

If truth be told, the average person probably does eat a little too much bread when you add up the 2 slices at breakfast, the 3 or 4 at lunch, and maybe the odd extra piece here and there.

But it's not the bread itself that contributes to excessive weight gain, rather the calories from it.

Depending on what type you buy, a slice will have 70 to 100 calories; so 8 slices a day could be a whopping 800 calories.

It might do you some good to switch your sandwich for a salad occasionally, or have Greek yoghurt instead of jam on toast at breakfast, but in isolation, bread will not make you fat and it doesn't make sense to remove it or any other wholegrains from your diet.

What's more, there is a large volume of research[17] which shows that there are many health benefits to be had from including whole grains in the diet. These include improved blood lipid profile, glucose control, cardiovascular health and reduced risk of stroke.[18][19] There have even been studies showing that removing bread from your diet can hinder your fat loss![20]

In one study, two groups were placed on a low-calorie diet. One group was allowed to eat bread, the other wasn't. After 16 weeks, the bread-eaters had a greater compliance with the diet with fewer dropouts!

TAKE-HOME HABIT

Grains have benefits. The unwarranted removal of grains from the diet can be time-consuming, reduce the enjoyment of food and make eating a balanced diet inconvenient, so don't make healthy eating harder than it needs to be.

8. CARDIOACCELERATE YOUR PROGRESS

You've probably not heard of cardioacceleration training before but it's a fantastic way to add in a cardio component to a weights workout and rev up the calories you burn in the process.

All you have to do is include 30–60 seconds of high intensity cardio between your sets of weight lifting. Let's say you're doing an upper body workout and you've just done a set of shoulder presses. Rather than just sitting around, playing on your phone or people-watching, you bust out 30–60 seconds of cardio like burpees, mountain climbers, star jumps, running on the spot, and so on.

You get the benefits of a HIIT workout and a resistance training workout at the same time! In sciency terms, this is called 'concurrent training', and there is evidence that shows that it's the bee's knees.

In one study in the *Journal of Strength and Conditioning Research*,[21] participants who performed cardioacceleration between sets experienced greater increases in lower body strength, lower body endurance, fat-free mass and flexibility compared with the group who didn't do cardioacceleration!

It gets better. A similar study,[22] by the same authors, found that cardioacceleration also rapidly reduces the duration participants experience DOMS (Delayed Onset Muscle Soreness). DOMS is the aching feeling you get in your muscles after a hard workout or if you start a new sport or exercise that you've either not done before or not done in a while. Think walking upstairs after a leg workout.

» Putting it into practice

- Firstly, I wouldn't do this in every workout; I would perhaps only include it on occasion to mix things up and only on an upper body day. I wouldn't want to give up my precious rest periods between squats and deadlifts in favour of 30 seconds of burpees.

- Secondly, you have to make sure that it doesn't impact on the quality of your workout or increase your risk of injury. Sure, it can be a great way to increase calorie burn, but if it comes at the cost of you lifting less total volume in your workout because you're gassed, then it's not going to be worth it.

TAKE-HOME HABIT

Cardioacceleration can be a great way to get the benefits of a HIIT workout and resistance training in one, but don't go overboard. Incorporating it a couple of times per week is going to increase calorie expenditure.

9. BIN THE FAT-BURNING SUPPLEMENTS

'Fat-burning' supplements sound like an amazing idea.

Pop a few capsules and your metabolism will be supercharged and the fat will melt off you like wax under a flame.

Unfortunately, the 'fat-burning' benefits of the most popular ingredients found in these pills are grossly exaggerated.

Let's look at some of the most popular ones.

Green Tea Extract
I explain in Go Easy on the Green Tea (page 60) why green tea isn't worth drinking unless you actually enjoy the flavour. The metabolism-boosting properties are fairly non-existent, but you'll still find that it's one of the main ingredients found in fat-burning supplements.

CLA
Conjugated Linoleic Acid, or CLA for short, is often touted as a great supplement if fat loss is your goal. CLA has been shown to increase fat burning by 60–80% in mice.[23]

Does this apply to you? I'm afraid not. In humans the results are so insignificant that it's unlikely to make any difference to your physique. One study showed that 3.4g daily CLA supplementation for a year didn't make any difference at all.[24]

L-carnitine

L-carnitine often appears in fat-burning supplement blends, but some folk also take it on its own. As you probably imagined from the theme of this chapter, it's not really going to do anything for you. One 8-week study in moderately obese women found that taking 2g per day didn't contribute to weight loss.[25]

There is an exception. If you're over 100 years old, then it's good news. One study in centenarians found that it did actually help reduce body fat and increase lean mass (among other benefits),[26] but for the majority of us it's not worth it.

TAKE-HOME HABIT

In reality, most fat-burners do two things: they give you a caffeine boost and mildly supress your appetite. Both of these can be achieved by drinking more coffee and eating some more protein.

10. CAPITALISE ON COMPOUND LIFTS

A compound or multi-joint lift is one where you recruit several muscle groups to perform the exercise.

These lifts can help you get more done in the gym, in less time!

Deadlifts, bench presses, lunges and leg presses are all examples of compound lifts you might be familiar with. The opposite of a compound lift is an isolation lift, like a dumbbell curl. The movement happens in one place; in the case of a dumbbell curl, it's at the elbow.

If you're looking to burn fat, embrace the compound lifts.

» **Here's why**

- Firstly, because you're using more than one muscle group, you generally burn more calories doing compound lifts compared with isolation lifts.[27] Think how much harder you must work to do a squat compared with a leg extension. Both exercises are targeting the quadriceps, but when you squat you use your quadriceps, hamstrings and glutes, you use your core and back to maintain an upright position, and you use your arms to grip onto the bar or dumbbells.

- Compound lifts also stimulate more blood flow and increase your heart rate more than isolation lifts and you get a slightly bigger increase in EPOC, which is short for Excess Post-Exercise Oxygen Consumption. Often informally known as the 'afterburn', this is when your body continues to burn calories after exercise to help repair your body and return it to a resting state.

(cont.)

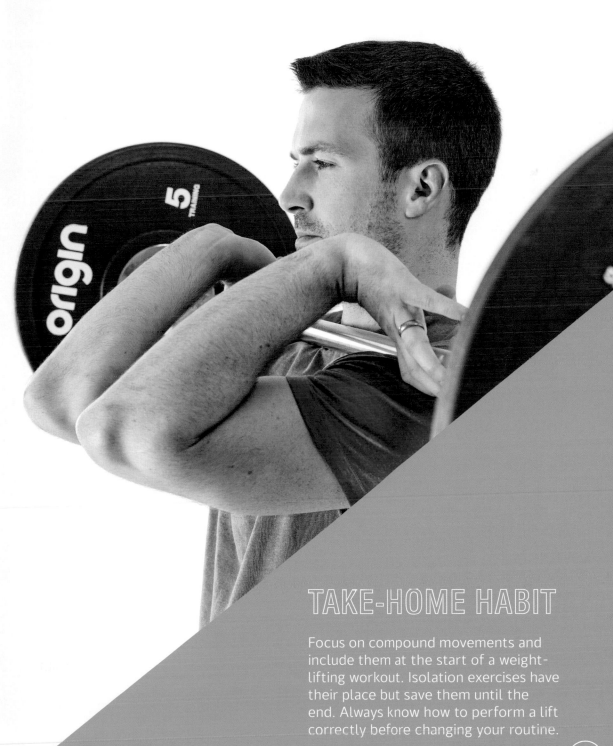

TAKE-HOME HABIT

Focus on compound movements and include them at the start of a weight-lifting workout. Isolation exercises have their place but save them until the end. Always know how to perform a lift correctly before changing your routine.

CAPITALISE ON COMPOUND LIFTS

- Another benefit of compound lifts, unknown to many, is that they are some of the best abdominal exercises you could do. Yup, I bet you didn't know that squatting and pull-ups are actually fantastic for your core. When squatting, you fire-up your abdominals to keep your back upright and your core tight. For pull-ups, your abs are required to keep your body upright and in line with the bar.

- The nature of compound lifts means that you can target various muscle groups more frequently if you train a couple of times per week. This is been shown numerous times[28] to be more effective than just training a body part once per week. If you train twice per week, rather than doing an upper body workout one day then a lower body the next, switch to doing a whole body workout each time and you'll get greater muscle recruitment over the week.

11. HACK YOUR MEAL PREP WITH GADGETS

Digital scales

If you don't have digital scales already then they should be your number-one purchase, especially if you're tracking your macros or keeping a food diary. It's important to measure certain foods, especially calorie-dense ones like nuts, to make sure you don't eat too much. For the first few weeks at least, weigh all the foods to give you an idea of what 30g nuts, for example, looks like; it's likely to be less than you think, unfortunately. These ones are top-rated and reasonably priced: weightlossbook.co.uk/scales

Thermal food flask

Don't have access to a microwave at work to heat your lunch? No problem. This Thermos® food flask is fantastic! It's wider than a typical flask and perfect for keeping meals piping hot so you can have a tasty, hot meal for lunch instead of a soggy, cold stew: weightlossbook.co.uk/flask

Meal prep bag

This is the ultimate cool bag. These were originally popularised by bodybuilders who were slaves to eating chicken, broccoli and brown rice 9 times per day. Nowadays, they're a great option for people who don't have access to a fridge at work or do a lot of travelling with their job. There are plenty of compartments to keep your meals cold, room to store your gym kit and water bottles, and they're durable, too: weightlossbook.co.uk/bag

TAKE-HOME HABIT

Adding a couple of nifty gadgets to your kitchen, like the ones mentioned here, will help make meal prep easier.

12. GET INTO SLOW COOKING

Slow cookers are a must-have if you want to win at meal prep.

Throw your food into your slow cooker in the morning and head off to work. Walk in the door 8 hours later and you've got a delicious pot of rich, meaty, juicy food to feed the whole family.

How can this help you lose weight? By ensuring that you can never use the 'I don't have time to cook healthy meals' excuse. Plus, they're an easy way to cook up big batches of healthy meals and freeze them in portions.

What's more, food that's cooked slowly at a low temperature tends to retain more vitamins, and serving the dish with the gravy it was cooked in helps increase its nutritional content.

Slow cookers can be great for veg-averse people, too. It's very easy to throw a tonne of different vegetables into the slow cooker. Because the veg is cooked with the meat, they take on a delicious rich, meaty flavour. If the thought of boiled carrots doesn't float your boat, throw them into your favourite stew in the slow cooker and the flavours will transform.

Another benefit is that it's a really cost-effective method of cooking too! Compared to an electric oven, they use considerably less energy. Your oven uses around 4,000 watts of power each hour it runs. Slow cookers, on the other hand, use just 300 watts.

'Yeah, but if I have to cook my meat for hours on end, surely that can't be cheaper?'
Wrong.

Let's say you've got a hunk of beef brisket that would take 2 hours to roast in an oven but 6 hours in a slow cooker. Even with the longer cooking time, the slow cooker would use a total of 1,800 watts. The oven would use 8,000 watts. Since electricity is priced by usage, using a slow cooker is much greener and cheaper!

Another way they save money is that you can get away with using cheaper, tougher cuts of meat that you wouldn't normally use if you were in a hurry.

When you cook meat on a low temperature for several hours, the collagen and connective tissues have a chance to soften, which tenderises the meat. Slow cooking brings out the best in their flavour and it can transform cheap cuts of meat into delicious, juicy chunks of meat that fall apart in your mouth.

Here's the most popular recipe from my ebook *The High Protein Handbook 4*.

Slow-Cooker Peanut Chicken
   1kg [2¼lb] chicken breast, diced
   1 onion, chopped
   2 clove garlic, crushed
   120g [½ cup] peanut butter
   1 tbsp cornflour [corn starch]
   400g [14oz] can of chopped tomatoes
   1 red chilli, deseeded
   2 tbsp lime juice
   1 tbsp curry powder
   2 tbsp soy sauce

Throw all of the ingredients into the slow cooker, cover and cook on low for 5 hours. Easy!

TAKE-HOME HABIT

Slow cookers are a fantastic way to win at meal prep. They save you money and hours in the kitchen.

13. AVOID EATING LIKE MY GRANDMA

You've never seen someone eat as fast as my grandma.
I'll just be putting the first forkful of food into my mouth and Janet's done already. She's the Usain Bolt of plate clearing; it's quite spectacular. If you think you could give her a run for her money, then this tip is going to be a winner for you...

Eat more slowly.

A LOT of research has been done on this. People who are fast eaters are generally heavier than people who take their time.[29] Other studies have shown that you can lose weight and reduce your overall calories, simply by reducing your eating speed.[30]

When you don't take my granny's approach to eating, your brain has more time to chat to your gut and receive key messages from your stomach and digestive track that lets it know that you're full.

It takes around 20 minutes from when you start eating before your brain receives these important messages. My granny could have eaten about 20 main courses in that time. When you slow down, your brain has a much better chance of letting you know when to stop and confirming that you don't need seconds.

So, how can you eat more slowly?

» Don't get distracted

As mention in Turn off the TV & Dine at the Table (page 94), when you're distracted, you'll eat more. Make sure you only eat meals at the table and not in front of the telly or computer.

» Eat with others

If you grab lunch with some friends or sit around the table with your family and chat, then you'll slow your eating speed down, too, compared with wolfing it down on your own.

» Set a 'chew-per-bite' goal

As strange as this sounds, increase the number of chews you do per bite, instead of swallowing down your food in one go like a duck.

» Put your fork and knife down

Think about what you're doing after each bite.

» Wait at least 20 minutes between courses

Be patient. As mentioned earlier, you need to allow time for the hunger signals to hit your brain. You might not need that pudding, after all.

TAKE-HOME HABIT

Slower eating will take a bit of time to get familiar with and at first it will seem very unnatural, but the science shows that it is a simple way to cut back on your calories and help your weight loss.

14. MAKE A PLAN, NOT JUST A WISH

'I'd like to lose weight.'
'I want to tone up.'
'I'm going to start eating better.'

These are aims, dreams and ideas. They're not goals. Goals can be measured. Goals have quantifiable outcomes. Goals can be tracked. Goals are dreams with deadlines!

Before you go any further into this book, you need to write down exactly why you're reading this book and what you want to happen as a result!

I love the SMART framework for setting goals:
Specific Measurable Attainable Realistic Time-Bound

Your weight loss goal needs to fit that criteria if you actually want it to happen.

Specific
Exercising more is not specific, neither is doing more steps. Going to the gym twice per week or hitting 10,000 steps per day is.

Measurable
If you can't measure it, you can't track it. Getting fitter isn't measurable. Running 5k in 30 seconds faster than you could do now is. Eating better isn't measurable. Eating protein at breakfast (see Pile on the Protein at Breakfast on page 20) or only eating at the table (see Turn off the TV & Dine at the Table on page 94) is.

Attainable
If you do no exercise at the moment, committing to going to the gym 5 times per week is setting yourself up to fail. Swapping all chocolate in your diet for fruit would also be fairly futile. However, going to the gym twice per week or only having chocolate at the weekend would be far more attainable goals.

Realistic

Thanks to the garbage on social media and in the magazines you might think that losing 6lb in 6 days or dropping a stone in a week is realistic. Sure, if you want to starve yourself, feel like death and gain it all back again, go ahead. A much more realistic target is to aim for a loss of 1–2lb a week.[31]

Time-Bound

You need a date. Open-ended goals can be postponed, the healthy habits can go on hold and you'll be more likely to just jack it all in. Short-term goals are the business. Don't stress about where you want to be in 6 months, that's ages away, stick to 30-day 'sprints' instead.

TAKE-HOME HABIT

Weight-loss goals should be SMART ones and focus on short blocks of around 30 days at a time.

15. YEARN TO BE A YOGI AT HOME

Increased flexibility, increased muscle strength, improved energy and vitality, protection from injury, improved athletic performance, and importantly for us – weight loss.

Yoga seems to be the ultimate activity if you want to improve your all-round health and wellbeing along with your waistline.

One study of 80 obese males found that after 14 weeks of yoga, participants experienced a reduction in weight, body mass index and skin fold thickness.[32]

So how exactly does yoga help you lose weight? Researchers at the NIH Clinical Centre found 5 main reasons for how it can help you on your quest to a trimmer tummy.[33]

- Yoga can result in an increase in mindful eating, changes in food choices, and decreased emotional and/or stress eating.

- The culture of yoga can aid weight loss in that yoga teachers and more advanced yoga practitioners often serve as role models for healthy behaviours and there is a strong sense of support among the yoga community.

- The physiological changes from yoga include increased muscle tone, increased strength and changes in metabolism that can enhance weight loss.

- Yoga can promote a shift in mindset away from weight loss and towards health, spirituality, increased mindfulness and focus, improved mood and emotional stability, reduced stress, and increased self-esteem and self-acceptance.

- A yoga regime is often more enjoyable to adhere to in comparison to traditional 'restriction diets' which can make it more enjoyable.

Yoga is even more accessible than ever.

You don't even need to go to a class. There are a multitude of free yoga classes online and plenty of mobile apps that you can download to help you go from being a Stiff Steve to a Flexible Fred in no time.

TAKE-HOME HABIT

Yoga may be an easy and enjoyable habit to improve your overall health and reduce your waistline.

16. FAST-TRACK FAT-BURNING WITH A FAST

Intermittent fasting (IF) is quite popular on the fitness scene and it's gone mainstream thanks to books like *The 5:2 Diet Book* and *Eat Stop Eat*.

If you're not sure what it entails, quite simply, fasting is when you limit the amount of food you eat for a given period, followed by a period of normal eating.

Does it work?
Yes. In one systematic review, IF followers lost 3–8% of their body weight over 3–24 weeks.[34] Not only that, but fasting has been shown to decrease blood sugar levels, reduce oxidative stress and blood pressure and improve cholesterol.[35]

How would I do it?
There are many ways in which people can approach IF. There's the alternate-day fast, in which you restrict your calories every other day, a fast once in every seven days, or a fast every third day. However, the two most popular approaches are the 16:8 method and the 5:2 method. In the 16:8 method, you spend 16 hours a day fasting and you have an eating window of 8 hours. The 5:2 method is when you have 5 'normal' eating days and 2 days on 500 calories.

What are the disadvantages?
A serious problem for many, not surprisingly, is hunger, and that can hamper adherence.[36] If you find that you're susceptible to the 'hanger' demons, then fasting probably isn't for you and a more frequent eating pattern is probably the smarter choice.

It can also hamper your training, too. If you train first thing in the morning, you haven't eaten since the night before and you're not going to eat until midday, then you might not feel you have that much energy. However, you can be smart and move your training timetable around so that you hit the gym after you've had a feed.

Now, although fasting sounds like it's the cure to all dieting woes, you've got to understand that the reason why it works is simply because when you shorten your 'eating window' you're likely to consume fewer calories as a result.

It's not really down to any mystical metabolism-boosting or hormone-optimising wizardry, it's because you'll eat less.

TAKE-HOME HABIT

Fasting could be a fantastic and simple way for you to decrease your calorie intake. If you find that you're able to follow it without becoming a hangry demon, then power and praise to you!

17. CHANGE UP YOUR COFFEES

Another one of the fat-loss tips that the guru fit-pros love to tell you, is that regardless of what kind of coffee you drink, you should swap it for a green tea or an Americano. If they're feeling lenient, they'll let you have an Americano with skimmed milk... How fun...

I'm all on board with the idea of limiting the number of calories that you drink; it's generally far more satiating if you eat your calories instead of drinking them. For some people, some simple changes to their coffees can boost their fat loss.

Don't worry, we're not going to go to extremes. If you drink quite a lot of calorie-heavy coffees over the course of a week, ditching them in favour of green tea is never going to last (green tea is hugely over-rated as a fat-burner anyway – see page 60).

» Here's an idea

Make simple changes like swapping from whole milk to semi-skimmed, pick a sugar-free syrup instead of the sugary sweet ones, have 1 sugar instead of 2, pick a smaller size takeaway coffee than usual, ditch the whipped cream toppings, etc. You get the idea.

You don't need to just go straight for the absolute lowest of the low-calorie coffees like a skimmed Americano either. Look at this: you can get a 'grande' (that's the 2nd largest size for those of us not inclined to speak Starbucks®) cappuccino for only 115 calories. That's one-fifth of the calories in a whopper of the same-size white chocolate mocha.

You may have seen the fitness craze where people ruin a tasty cup of coffee by adding in a stick of butter and coconut oil. Yes, you read that correctly, people do that and claim it's fat burning. Now, if you're this far through the book and you think a 500-calorie cup of coffee is fat burning, then you've not been paying attention.

Successful and lasting fat loss will be down to you adopting healthier habits that you can follow in the long run. It's also crucial that you actually like the food and drinks that you're going to be replacing or modifying in the quest to a trimmer waistline.

So let's not go too extreme, ok?

TAKE-HOME HABIT

Ditch the fancy coffees that are laden with calories and go for a simple coffee with milk or choose the 'skinny' version of your favourite drink instead.

18. SKIP THE SIT-UPS & PERFECT THE PLANKS

If you're trying to burn fat, sit-ups are probably one of the most useless exercises you could do!

Yet you see so many people doing them in the gym in their quest for a flatter stomach or tighter tummy.

» Here's why

You can't burn fat from a specific body part by exercising it. This is called the 'spot reduction myth'. Doing triceps exercises won't get rid of fat from the arms, working on the glutes won't burn fat from the bum, and sit-ups, crunches or any abdominal exercise for that matter, won't burn fat from the belly.[37]

Unfortunately, you can't decide where you're going to lose body fat from. If you're in a calorie deficit and you're following the tips in this book, your body will gradually shed its fat from most places where it's stored. Some folk will see it go from the face more quickly; others will notice their waist coming in; others still will find it goes from their bum first. We're all different and how our body fat is distributed, and where we lose it from first, varies significantly.

From an exercise perspective, although there are no 'fat-burning exercises' per se, the ones that generally burn the most calories are compound exercises, which we discussed on page 30.

Although sit-ups don't have much, if any, effect on your abdominal fat, they do have some merit in that they will help to strengthen your core and improve muscular endurance. However, there are better core exercises that you could be doing instead.

Leg raises and rollouts are both very challenging. If you struggle to do a rollout with an abs wheel, you can start off by doing it on an exercise ball. It's a good idea to include some isometric exercises too. Isometric exercises are done in 'static positions', rather than being dynamic (when you do a lot of movement). Isometric abdominal exercises include the plank, side plank and bird dogs.

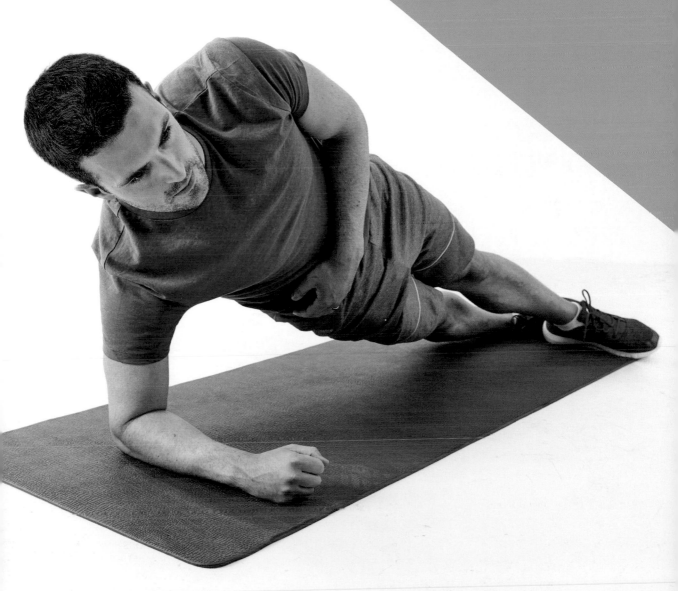

TAKE-HOME HABIT

Skip the sit-ups if you're trying to get leaner and focus on compound exercises and cardio instead. If you do want to develop a stronger core, consider some of the more effective alternatives.

To see video demonstrations for the abs exercises mentioned, head to weightlossbook.co.uk/resources

19. IGNORE THE MEAL-TIMING MYTHS

Healthy eating can be a confusing subject and meal timing is a classic example of one of its tricky aspects.

Trying to find out the facts about what to eat, when to eat and how much to eat can be a frustrating experience.

Myth #1

Small, frequent meals speed up your metabolism.
You must eat every two hours to boost metabolism.
You've heard that one before, haven't you? Research actually shows[38] us that it's your total energy intake vs energy output that influences your body composition, not how many meals you've eaten. How often you should eat is really down to you. If you're a three-meals-a-day person and you're always hungry, I would consider adding in a mid-morning and mid-afternoon snack – perhaps some fruit, nuts or yoghurt. This doesn't 'boost metabolism', but it will help reduce hunger and it may prevent overeating at your bigger meals.

Myth #2

Carbs eaten at night (after 6PM) are more likely to be stored as fat.

This is probably one of the most popular myths out there. Thankfully, carbohydrates eaten after 6PM don't suddenly zoom to your waistline and cause you to gain weight.[39] How *much* you eat over the course of your day dictates body composition, not specifically when you eat. Sure, eating fewer carbohydrates in the evening could help you lose weight, but it's probably because you've reduced your total intake, not because you stopped eating after 6PM. See page 157.

Myth #3

You must neck a protein shake straight after a workout.

Guess what? Research shows[40] there is no significant difference in body composition changes between people who chug a protein shake right after training and those who wait two to three hours after training to eat.

TAKE-HOME HABIT

Don't sweat the small stuff, like how many times you eat per day or what time you eat. Eat when and how often you want!

20. MASTER MACROS WITH FLEXIBLE DIETING

Flexible dieting is the concept whereby you can essentially eat any food you choose so long as it fits within your individual calorie allowance and macronutrient (protein, carbs and fat) targets.

You can eat 'good' food 80% of the time, for example, meaning nutrient-dense, filling, fibrous 'healthy' foods (although that term is subjective). And the remaining 20% of the time you'll have leeway to include some less nutritious foods like ice cream, sweets, crisps, chocolate, etc into your macronutrient allowance.

You may have also heard the acronym IIFYM (If It Fits Your Macros), which is the same thing, although that term has some stigma associated with it whereby people assume followers of the IIFYM protocol just try and eat as much junk as possible... so long as 'it fits your macros, bro'.

Unfortunately, despite what you may have seen posted on Instagram, flexible dieting isn't just a challenge to see how much weight you can lose simply by slamming sweets, chocolate bars and fast food. You can certainly include these things in your macro allowance, but you may find it hard to hit your fibre target and you might find you'll go hungry if you've assigned 80% of your total calories to one monstrous meal.

The good news is that science supports flexible dieting for long-term weight-loss success.

'Rigid dieting strategies reported symptoms of an eating disorder, mood disturbances, and excessive concern with body size/shape. Flexible dieting strategies were not highly associated with BMI, eating disorder symptoms, mood disturbances, or concerns with body size.'[41]

'... rigid eating behaviours lead to food cravings thereby hampering long-term weight maintenance. Indeed, people with flexible control strategies have been found to be more successful in long-term weight maintenance.'[42]

To get started with flexible dieting you'll need to work out your calorie, protein, fat and carbohydrate targets. This tool will do all the hard work for you: weightlossbook.co.uk/resources

TAKE-HOME HABIT

With flexible dieting, you're likely to follow an 80/20 split. Find a balance that works for you, once you've figured out your macro targets.

21. SHED POUNDS WITH FRIENDS

Teamwork makes the dream work. It's no different if you're trying to lose weight.

'Study participants reported significantly greater weight loss, health and fitness results when they had the support of family and friends.'[43]

'Study participants who actively enlisted the social support of 3 or more friends experienced 176% greater long-term success with their exercise and nutrition program than those who tried to do it on their own.'[44]

If you want to lose weight, and keep it off, you shouldn't go it alone – you've got to get some others in your team.

The first step is to tell someone about your goals. This makes them real and they'll hold you accountable. If you try and go it alone, nobody is there to help pick you up if you fall off the bandwagon or to offer praise when you succeed.

It's always easier and more fun with a buddy. Let's say you've read Visualise the Body You Want (page 212) and you've committed to going for a walk every lunchtime as you work towards hitting your 10,000 steps every day. Some days it's going to rain, some days you'll be busy, some days you simply won't have the motivation to get up and go outside. Add a 'walking buddy' into the equation and you've got a different scenario entirely. If you've got a colleague doing the same, who you walk with every lunchtime, they're going to be there to hold you accountable. Are you really going to let them walk outside in the rain on their own?

**Apparently, we are the average of the 5 people
we spend the most time with.**

If all your family are overweight, if you only hang out with
friends over food, if your colleagues spend most of the day
sitting at a desk then in front of the TV at home, then the odds
of succeeding are stacked against you.

Thanks to the internet and social media, you can easily find
a group of like-minded folk in the same boat as you who are
encountering the same struggles. What's more, they want you
to join them. They want their social support group to grow as
much as you want to find one!

TAKE-HOME HABIT

Build a team, share your goals, find a
tribe. P.S. There's a space for you if you
want to join our Fat Loss Inner Circle:
weightlossbook.co.uk/join

22. REFUEL WITH A REFEED DAY

The pros down the gym love to talk about their 'cheat days' and 'cheat meals'. When you eat nothing but chicken, broccoli and brown rice, it's no surprise that come the weekend you're itching to eat something with some flavour!

If you follow a flexible dieting approach, as described in Master Macros with Flexible Dieting (page 50), this doesn't happen. As you have the leeway to incorporate tastier, less nutritionally sound foods into your normal eating routine to help minimise cravings and to make dieting considerably more tolerable, you don't need to have a huge, unregulated feed composed of mainly junk foods, in the hope that it boosts metabolism and gives you a welcome break from dieting.

I recommend a controlled 'Single-Day Refeed'.

On a refeed day, you bring your calories back up to maintenance level, fat drops a little and carbohydrate increases significantly. You would include a refeed once per week. Some folk do it at the weekend to give them something to look forward to; others have a refeed the day before their hardest training day.

The single-day refeed may help to prevent certain metabolic adaptations, to give you a physiological boost. It should also improve training performance for a few days afterwards and will help to minimise loss of muscle.

What are 'metabolic adaptations'?

When you're in a calorie deficit and you're dieting, you will experience certain metabolic adaptations.[45] For example, this may include adaptive thermogenesis (your resting metabolic rate decreases), increased mitochondrial efficiency (your body becomes more effective at exercising with fewer calories) and hormonal alterations that favour decreased energy expenditure, decreased satiety, and, unfortunately, increased hunger.

Remember that you must still track everything you eat on your refeed day!

TAKE-HOME HABIT

If you're following a flexible dieting approach, consider including a refeed day once a week.

23. NOTCH UP YOUR NEAT THE EASY WAY

NEAT is the largest contributor to your overall calorie expenditure, outside 'formal exercise', that you have probably never heard of.

It's short for Non-Exercise Activity Thermogenesis and it is the calories you burn by fidgeting, walking, standing, coughing, waving your arms around, giving high fives and basically any form of energy expended that isn't sleeping, eating or exercise.

It's kind of a big deal.

NEAT could result in an increase of hundreds more calories burned per day depending on someone's weight and level of activity.[46]

The longer and longer you stay in a calorie deficit, your body becomes more efficient and uses less energy for everyday tasks and NEAT declines. This called 'metabolic adaptation'.[47] For example, you fidget less to conserve energy and you burn fewer calories in a workout, too.[48]

A decrease in NEAT is often one of the main reasons why people stop losing weight and hit a plateau. If it drops significantly, it may mean that you're no longer in a calorie deficit because your maintenance calories have dropped as a result.

Are you following?

It can be quite easily fixed.

What you need to do is to try and get your NEAT back up again! Think about going for some walks and stand at your desk for a while, as we discuss in Stand More to Burn More (page 186). You could park a little further from work, take the dog an extra loop round the block, take the stairs rather than the lift, get off the bus earlier, do some bodyweight exercises when watching TV. All of these activities, whilst not seeming that significant in isolation, will add up.

TAKE-HOME HABIT

If you're trying to lose weight, it's crucial that you keep on top of your NEAT and adopt habits and routines that will keep it high and recognise that the longer you're in a calorie deficit, the harder and harder it will be.

24. POWER UP YOUR PROTEIN WITH A SHAKE

Do I need to drink protein shakes?

Quite simply, no, you don't need to drink a protein shake. You can get all the protein you need from protein-rich whole foods like poultry, beef, beans, pulses, fish and dairy.

However, the occasional use of a protein supplement can help you to hit your protein targets if you have a higher requirement or if you struggle to consume a sufficient quantity of protein from whole foods.

Protein powders can be an easy, tasty and cost-effective method of ensuring you get enough protein in your diet, but they're certainly not essential.

What are the different kinds of protein powders?

The most popular form of protein on the market is called whey protein. Whey is a bi-product from making cheese and it has a very high biological value (BV). A high BV means it is easily digested and a large proportion of it is absorbed by the body.

There are other powders that are popular with people who follow a plant-based diet, such as brown rice protein or soy protein. However, these sources have a lower BV score and are less readily available in the shops. Some people take a casein protein supplement, but I haven't seen a convincing volume of research to suggest casein is superior to whey, although some research suggests that it may be more filling if you're trying to lose weight.

When should I take protein after a workout?

Contrary to gym-lore, there isn't a rapid urgency to consume protein immediately after a workout. The post-exercise 'anabolic window' is an often misunderstood subject.

Research in the *Journal of the International Society of Sports Nutrition* (JISSN)[49] suggests that the window of opportunity lasts considerably longer than 45 minutes. For most people, consuming a 25g+ serving of protein (any type of quality protein source, not specifically a shake) within 3 hours of exercise will be sufficient to stimulate the muscle recovery process (known as muscle protein synthesis, or MPS). In practical terms, this means if you exercise before lunch, make sure your lunch contains a suitable serving of protein. The same rule applies if you're working out before dinner, before breakfast, and so on.

There is also evidence[50] to suggest that consuming around 40g of 'pre-sleep protein' is an effective dietary strategy to improve overnight muscle protein synthesis and improve training recovery. So you might want to have a protein-rich snack shortly before going to bed. This could be a wholefood option or simply a protein shake, or perhaps some protein powder mixed with oats to make a protein porridge.

TAKE-HOME HABIT

You don't need a protein shake, but it can be a handy supplement to help you reach a higher protein target.

25. GO EASY ON THE GREEN TEA

Losing weight is something that many people want to experience – and the faster it happens (and the less strenuous effort involved), the better. It's no surprise, then, that anything that claims to be 'fat burning' will always have a ready market!

Enter the humble cup of green tea.

Green tea is rich in antioxidants called catechins. The one that receives the most attention, and is often reported to be the fat-burner or metabolism-booster, is called epigallocatechin gallate or EGCG for short. Before we go any further, it's important to note that a regular sized cup of green tea will contain around 50mg EGCG.

In one study[51] looking at the effects of catechin-enriched green tea on body composition, the group who drank the highest concentration of catechins in their green tea (886mg) lost 1.2kg more than the other groups in 90 days. However, that's the equivalent of 18 cups of green tea per day!

In 2012, a meta-analysis (this is a big study of other studies) examined 18 studies on the effect of green tea on weight loss involving 1,945 participants.[52]

Here's the conclusion:
'Green tea preparations appear to induce a small, statistically non-significant weight loss in overweight or obese adults. Because the amount of weight loss is small, it is not likely to be clinically important. Green tea had no significant effect on the maintenance of weight loss.'

The bottom line is that green tea may result in a tiny amount of weight loss but it's very insignificant.

Secondly, the amount you would have to drink for it to have even the slightest impact on your waistline is far greater than what you would happily drink in a day anyway.

TAKE-HOME HABIT

If you like green tea, that's fine, but don't force yourself to drink it because you think it's 'fat burning'.

26. TAKE THE 28-DAY PRESS-UP CHALLENGE

Press-ups are probably one of the best, if not the most popular, of all body weight exercises. You need zero equipment and they recruit a host of muscle groups including your chest, arms, shoulders and abdominals.[53]

There are plenty of variations, too. You can alter your body angle and do incline press-ups (when your hands are above your feet), decline are when your hands are below your feet, you can do close-grip, which puts more emphasis on your triceps, you can do single arm, you can add a clap, the list goes on.

Before we get into the challenge, some key things to remember when doing a press-up: keep your hips in line with your shoulders, use your hands to really grip the floor, keep your elbows tight into the body (don't let them flare out to the sides) and don't let your lower back sag to the ground.

Once you've got the perfect press-up position, let's start the challenge. The goal is to improve your technique, increase strength, muscular endurance and perhaps even to build a little muscle.

(cont.)

TAKE-HOME HABIT

Press-ups are a fantastic upper body exercise that help you to get stronger and develop your pushing power.

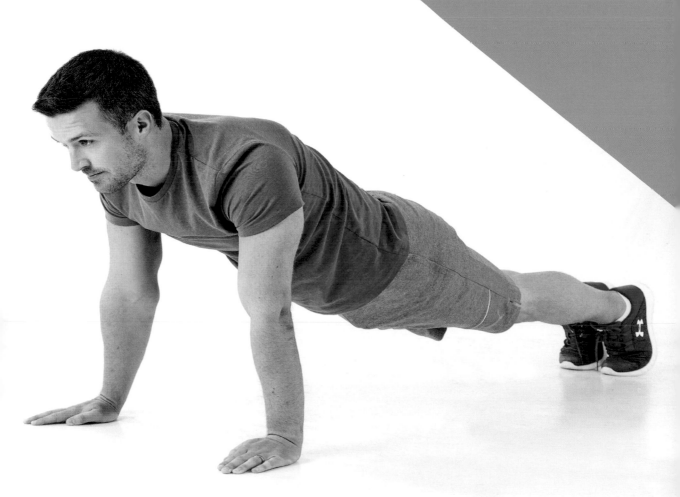

TAKE THE 28-DAY PRESS-UP CHALLENGE

Day 1 – **5**	Day 8 – **7/7/5**	Day 15 – **8/8/8**	Day 22 – **5/5/5/5/5**
Day 2 – **7**	Day 9 – **15**	Day 16 – **5/10/15**	Day 23 – **10/12/15**
Day 3 – **5/5***	Day 10 – **10/7/5/3**	Day 17 – **15/15**	Day 24 – **10/10/10**
Day 4 – **7/5**	Day 11 – **7/7/7**	Day 18 – **20**	Day 25 – **20/15/10/5**
Day 5 – **7/7**	Day 12 – **10/10**	Day 19 – **15/12/10**	Day 26 – **15/15/12**
Day 6 – **7/5/3**	Day 13 – **10/8/6/4**	Day 20 – **5/10/15/20**	Day 27 – **25**
Day 7 – **rest**	Day 14 – **rest**	Day 21 – **rest**	Day 28 – **AMRAP****

*Do 5 reps, rest for a few moments, then do 5 more
**As many reps as possible

» Here's another varation
See how many press-ups you can do in one go on day 1 then for
the next 28 days you must do one more than the previous day.
Let's say you can do 10 on day 1, day 2 you aim for 11, day 3 you
go for 12 and so on.

» You could also take 3 'press-up breaks' per day.
At any three points throughout the day say after waking up,
at lunchtime and before bed you set yourself a set number of
press-ups that you have to complete.

27. TRUST IN TETRIS® TO CUT CRAVINGS

If you've got an old Gameboy lying around then you're onto a winner as a 2014 study[54] found that a few games of Tetris helped to reduce food cravings.

That's right. If you've got a food craving, one of the best things you can do is distract yourself.

Remember the tune, 'do do dodo doo do dooo dooo dooo...,' no? Just me then. I get it, you probably haven't played Tetris® in about 20 years and I'm quite surprised it was the game of choice used by the researchers, but the findings still stand true: video games and other types of distractions can help you eat less.

One study also reported that playing with some modelling clay helped reduce chocolate cravings.[55]

So how does it work? This type of distraction is called 'Elaborated Intrusion Theory (EI)' and it works because a visually based task (like playing a computer game) decreases craving and craving imagery.

Researchers at the University of Exeter have even created an app that works on the same principal and helps players to develop better food habits. The first round of results showed promise: after four 10-minute sessions, players ate around 220 calories less per day.[56]

TAKE-HOME HABIT

If you're prone to cravings, have some form of distraction at hand. For example, play a few games on your phone, browse Instagram and Facebook, watch a bit of Netflix, find something to take your mind off the food.

28. BURN FAT WITH A BODYWEIGHT CIRCUIT

If you want to do a workout but the thought of heading down to a sweaty gym is as appealing as eating a bag of nails, then you need look no further than a bodyweight workout.

You don't need a gym membership or equipment – you can do them in your own living room. A lot of exercises use multiple muscle groups and you can easily modify them to suit your goals and abilities.

When it comes to doing a bodyweight workout, most people often just randomly throw together some sit-ups, press-ups and maybe some burpees... and maybe some more sit-ups. There are hundreds of bodyweight exercises you can do and, as with any training approach, it's probably better for you to have a plan, rather than freestyling.

A plan will keep you on track, allow you to see and track your progress, and provide some inspiration so you don't just do the same exercises over and over again.

》 Here are a couple of sample bodyweight workouts you can try:

Workout #1
See how many rounds you can perform in 20 minutes
• 5 x burpees
• 5 x press-ups
• 5 x mountain climbers, each side
• 5 x tuck squat jumps
• 5 x lunges, each leg
• 5 x leg raises, 5 reps

Workout #2

Perform 15 seconds of each exercise then rest for 10 seconds before doing the next exercise. See how many rounds you can perform in 20 minutes.

- Star jumps (aka Jumping jacks)
- High knees
- Crunches
- Jumping split squats
- Press-ups
- Reverse crunches

Workout #3

See how many rounds you can perform in 20 minutes.

- 5 x pull-ups (you'll need a pull-up bar or make use of a climbing frame in a playground)
- 10 x press-ups
- 15 x squats

TAKE-HOME HABIT

If you don't do any exercise at the moment, try and incorporate one or two bodyweight workouts into your weekly routine.

29. BAN THE PROTEIN BARS & BREAKFAST BISCUITS

I started eating protein bars over 10 years ago when they were like solid blocks of cardboard that would suck all the moisture from your mouth and take a solid half hour to chomp your way though.

Because of that, I'm not really a fan. I can't quite erase those memories from my palate.

Thankfully, they have come on a long way since then and many of the popular chocolate manufacturers are turning their hands to pimping up their products with added protein.

But don't be fooled. Just because something has 'added protein' on the label doesn't mean it's a smart choice. Many of the popular protein bars have an extremely similar nutritional breakdown to that of a chocolate bar, with the exception of 20g more protein.

If you really want a chocolate bar, just eat a chocolate bar!

If you want some extra protein, eat some more chicken or have a glass of milk. Or make the protein smoothie in Pile on the Protein at Breakfast on page 20. It's going to be considerably tastier, cheaper and it won't seem like you're fooling yourself by trying to claim that you're not just having a chocolate bar.

However, it's a different story if you make your own protein bars. There are tonnes of tasty recipes online that don't have all the garbage added that many off-the-shelf varieties have. They're fresher, tastier and often pack far fewer calories.

On a similar note, another type of food that is a bit of a swizz is the breakfast biscuit. Once again, fancy-pants marketing would like to fool you into thinking that these are a smart way to start your day.

They're not.

They're pretty much like any other biscuit – they digest quickly, they're low in fibre, they don't fill you up and they're not very nutritious.

At breakfast, stick to the more filling staples like muesli, oats, natural yoghurt, eggs, fruit, wholegrains and so on.

TAKE-HOME HABIT

Off-the-shelf protein bars are not dissimilar to chocolate bars except they're more expensive and less tasty. If you do like the convenience of a protein bar, try making your own instead.

30. FILL UP ON FIBRE-RICH FOOD

Unfortunately, there is no such thing as a 'superfood', but fibre comes pretty close.

Folk who get plenty of dietary fibre appear to be at significantly lower risk of developing coronary heart disease, stroke, hypertension, diabetes, obesity, and certain gastrointestinal diseases.[57]

What's more, and the good news for you, is that a higher fibre intake has also been associated with a lower body weight.[58]

There are two types of fibre: soluble and insoluble.

As the name suggests, soluble fibre breaks down and dissolves in your digestive tract. Foods that are high in this type of fibre include oats, fruit, root vegetables and flax seeds. Insoluble fibre, like wholemeal bread, cereals, nuts and seeds, is the opposite – it doesn't dissolve in water and it helps other foods pass through your digestive tract more easily.

Recent government guidelines recommend adults aim for around 30g per day,[59] but the average person eats almost half of that at 18g per day.

If you're tracking your macronutrient (protein, carbohydrate and fat) targets on a dietary tracking app, then tracking your fibre intake is often a smart idea, too. This helps to ensure that your carbohydrate sources are more nutritious and filling and you are more likely to get your carbs from sweet potato and strawberries than from sweeties.

❱❱ Here are 10 of the most fibre-rich foods you can find

- Split peas
- Lentils
- Figs
- Black beans
- Butter beans [lima beans]
- Chickpeas [garbanzo beans]
- Chia seeds
- Avocados
- Butternut squash
- Raspberries

TAKE-HOME HABIT

Try to include several servings of fibre-rich foods per day. If you're tracking your macros, add your fibre target and aim for that, too.

31. PLUG IN A PODCAST & BE INSPIRED

Just like a slow cooker, I never really understood what a podcast was and why everyone kept on raving about them... Until I saw the light.

I'm now a huge fan.

Fast forward a couple of years and not only do I LOVE listening to podcasts but I also host one of the top-rated fitness podcasts in the UK too (you can listen to it here: weightlossbook.co.uk/podcast).

A podcast is generally a radio show on a specific subject that is released a couple of times a week. The reason they're so good is because you can get a serious amount of learning done when you're doing tasks that are normally fairly mundane: the commute, cleaning the house, cardio, the morning dog walk...

'How can they help you lose fat?' **I hear you ask.**

Take my podcast – 'The Food For Fitness Podcast' – for example. Each week I interview an expert from the field of nutrition, sport science, dietetics, mindset or strength and conditioning.

These experts really are at the top of their game. There have been Olympians, professors, best-selling authors, renowned conference speakers and world-class educators sharing their best fitness advice with you, for free.

There have been a million downloads, hundreds of 5* reviews and it was named in the top 5 fitness podcasts by *Men's Health* magazine.

There are loads of other great podcasts on fitness out there, too. Just go to your favourite podcast player and see what takes your fancy.

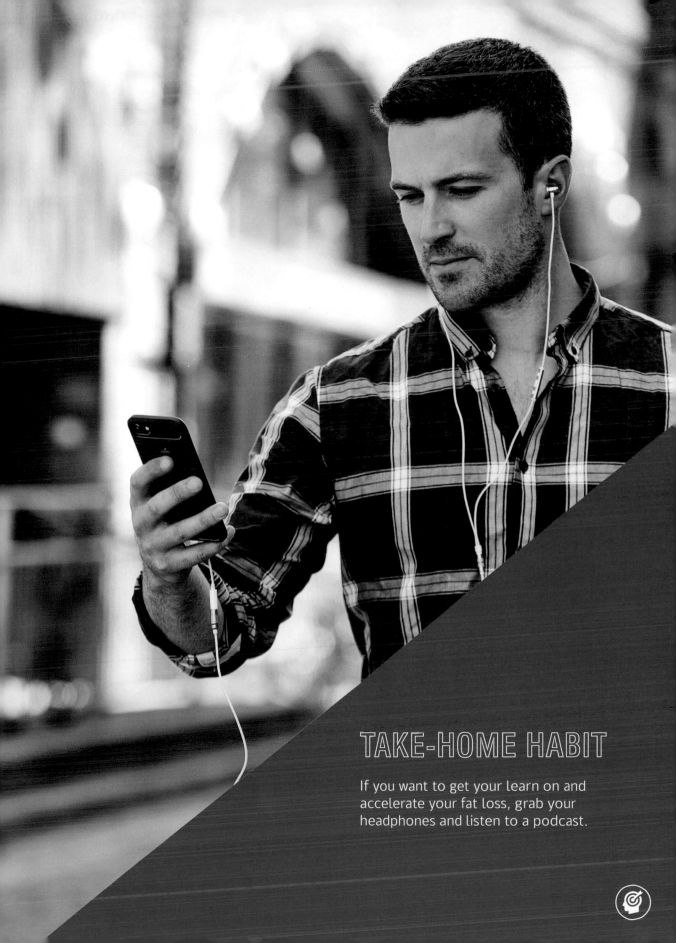

TAKE-HOME HABIT

If you want to get your learn on and accelerate your fat loss, grab your headphones and listen to a podcast.

32. FORGET THE 'FAT-BURNING ZONE'

If you've jumped onto any cardio machine in the gym, you will have seen the colourful graphics showing you the different heart rate zones. If you're exercising to get leaner, then there is a high chance you will have picked the programme that tries to keep your heart rate in the 'fat-burning zone' which is generally around 60–70% of your maximum heart rate.

Don't do this.

» Here's the science for you

Your body will burn different fuels depending on the exercise intensity. At a lower intensity, like in the fat-burning zone, your body will use fat for fuel. At a higher intensity, your body uses more carbohydrate[60].

Now, I know what you're thinking: 'So, why is this a bad thing?'

There are 24 hours in a day when you can burn fat; it's not limited to what happens in a 30-minute workout. If you're doing cardio as part of your routine, you want to focus on using it to help create or further your calorie deficit. This is when the real fat burning happens!

Look at it this way.

Option #1
You spend 30 minutes exercising in the 'fat-burning zone' and burn 200 calories.

Option #2
You spend 30 minutes exercising at a higher intensity and burn 350 calories.

Which do you think is going to be more effective over the course of a day? Exactly. Option 2.

So, yes, exercising at a lower intensity, like in the fat-burning zone, does burn calories and it may help you recover more easily if you've been doing sport or weights training but from a fat-loss perspective, it's not the most effective.

TAKE-HOME HABIT

If you're doing cardio to help you create your deficit, move out of the 'fat-burning zone' if you can, work at a higher intensity and burn more calories.

33. DROP THE JUICE DETOXES

Juice diets, cleanses, purges and reboots are a perpetual favourite of the short-term dieter. Often seen as a quick-fix weight-loss solution, their advocates would like to convince you that your body is bursting with toxins that need to leave.

The solution, they claim, lies in tall glasses brimming with fruits, vegetables and other 'superfoods'.

There are quite a few reasons why juicing is hugely overrated. For starters, any diet that causes you to make a monumental change in the way you eat or forces you to eliminate certain foods is unlikely to be sustainable.

Low-carb diets for someone who loves pasta, paleo diets for someone who devours dairy, vegetarian for a meat-lover and juice diets for the majority of us who eat solid food, are unlikely to result in long-term success.

If you completely exclude certain foods from your diet, you're going to experience cravings. You might manage to resist in the short-term, but at some point you'll break, you might binge and you'll reverse all your hard work.

Studies prove this.[61][62] Although no research has yet been done on the long-term effects of juice dieting, if you look at studies examining people who lose weight and keep it off, you'll see that they are the ones who generally take a more flexible approach to their food.

Another reason why you don't need to 'detox' is that your body is already doing this for you on a daily basis.

The human body has built-in toxin removers – they're called your liver and your kidneys. Any level of toxic material in the blood or elsewhere in the body that those organs cannot handle is far beyond anything a diet can cure.

There is also zero evidence that there are toxins in the body which build up over time and need to be purged with a special diet.

On a more positive note, juice diets aren't completely useless. They have some merit in that they can help you find new ways to get more fruit and veg into your diet, but you don't need to liquefy the food to achieve the same outcome.

Secondly, if you're a fussy eater and not a fan of vegetables, then blitzing up a vegetable smoothie can be a good way to eat more greens but it shouldn't be the only element in your diet.

TAKE-HOME HABIT

Skip the detoxes and focus on whole foods instead. Whole foods are more filling, nutritious and tastier than glasses of green goop!

34. CHALLENGE YOURSELF WITH CROSSFIT®

There is NOTHING else in existence that can claim responsibility for introducing more people to weightlifting than CrossFit. The good news is that there is way more to it than puking, pain and paleo.

'*CrossFit is constantly varied functional movements performed at high intensity. All CrossFit workouts are based on functional movements, and these movements reflect the best aspects of gymnastics, weightlifting, running, rowing and more.*' CrossFit Website[63]

It's the ultimate, varied workout.

Each day an official WOD 'Workout Of The Day' is posted on the website that can include anything from a 7km run to doing a certain number of gruelling squats for time, running backwards, and even doing handstand press-ups.

There are also the 'hero workouts' that are named after US serviceman who have passed away. The most famous being 'Murph', named after Lt. Michael P. Murphy, who was played by Mark Wahlberg in the 2003 film *Lone Survivor*.

Murph is a 1-mile run, 100 pull-ups, 200 press-ups, 300 squats then another 1 mile run... All while wearing a 20lb weighted vest.

There are thousands of CrossFit gyms, known as 'boxes', all over the world, that are packed with budding enthusiasts who become evangelised by the sport. As a result, the sense of camaraderie within the community is extremely strong and unlike anything seen in most other commercial gyms.

From a fat-loss perspective, CrossFit is fantastic. You get cardio, strength training, endurance and some serious calorie expenditure.[64]

Now there are some who don't like it and folk who say it's dangerous, largely due to some of the horrible videos posted online but a recent meta-analysis found that the injury rates with CrossFit is comparable with other exercise programmes with similar injury rates and health outcomes.[65]

I watched the docufilm 'Fittest On Earth: A Decade of Fitness', which follows some of the best CrossFit athletes in the world as they compete at the CrossFit Games, and I have to say I changed-up my training as a result, and it was fun; I liked it!

TAKE-HOME HABIT

If you've found that you like the idea of lifting weights but you've not been a fan of regular gym culture, or lack of community, then CrossFit might be for you.

35. FIGHT FAT WITH FRUIT

If there is one nutrition myth that grinds my gears more than almost any other, it's that you should avoid fruit if you're trying to fight the flab.

Fruit is fricking awesome.

Seriously though, avoid fruit?

» Here's the deal.

You will have heard of the 5-a-day guideline but new research suggests it may be better to aim for double that!

2.5 portions (200g) of fruit and veg per day is associated with a 16% reduced risk of heart disease, an 18% reduced risk of stroke, a 13% reduced risk of cardiovascular disease, 4% reduced risk of cancer and a 15% reduction in the risk of premature death.

How good is that?

But get this, 10 portions a day (800g) is associated with a 24% reduced risk of heart disease, a 33% reduced risk of stroke, a 28% reduced risk of cardiovascular disease, a 13% reduced risk of cancer, and a 31% reduction in premature deaths.[66]

Now, before you go and smash that entire punnet of grapes or munch a mountain of mango, remember that the rules of moderation still apply.

Fruit is not a free food. It still contains calories which means it will impact your body composition. Eat too much, move out of the calorie deficit and you won't lose weight.

The study mentioned above also looked at combined fruit and veg intake, not just fruit. My advice would be if you want to still reap the health benefits without a high calorie load, aim for a 60/40 veg to fruit split.

What about the sugars?

Yes, fruit does contain natural sugars but the vitamins, phytonutrients and fibre you'll get from fruit massively offset any potential negatives from the sugar content. Secondly, as part of a balanced diet, a small amount of sugar regardless of its source is unlikely to make any difference to your waistline.

TAKE-HOME HABIT

You certainly don't need to avoid fruit if you're trying to lose fat but, like any food, just be mindful of the calories and aim for a variety if you want to get a wide range of nutrients.

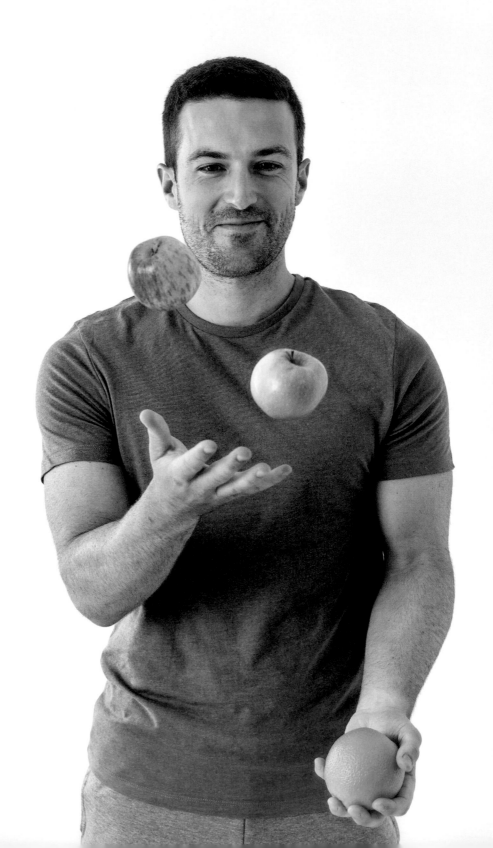

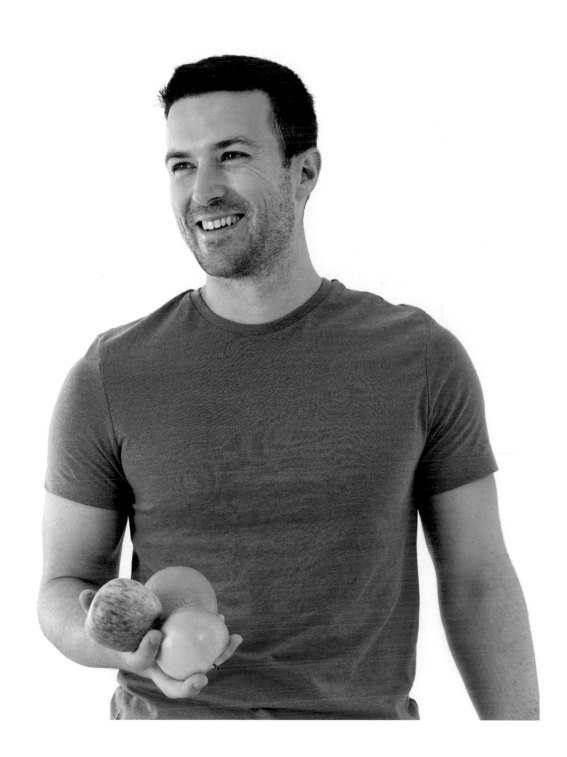

36. SPRUCE UP YOUR KIT & GET PLAYING

The beauty of sport is that it's one of the most fun ways to burn calories. You don't have to go to a gym to exercise. A tennis court, football pitch, running track, swimming pool, a road, volleyball court, etc can be your gym.

When people tell me they don't like going to a gym, I always ask them if they played sports when they were younger. When they say that they loved playing 5-a-side or they were on the netball team or they played badminton for their school, my next question is always, 'So, how can you get back into it?'

Unlike running on a treadmill, when you become fixated with the screen telling you how many calories you've burned and how long you've got left, with sport, you forget that you're exercising. It's fun. It's competitive. You're exercising with your mates. Time seems to fly by, and before you know it you're pouring with sweat and you've burned a tonne of calories in the process.

If you played sport when you were at school, or at university or before you had kids and you loved it, what's stopping you from going back to it? You probably already know some of your mates who are still playing; there are often corporate leagues that your work may be a part of, or a quick internet search will likely bring up a host of clubs close by that are dying for new members or players to join them.

Like anything worth doing in life, the hardest part is getting started. 'I bet they're all better than me.' 'I wouldn't be able to keep up.' 'I'll just let everyone down.' 'I don't want people to see how unfit I am.' That sort of defeatist, negative language is good for one thing: nothing.

Nobody cares if you're beginner.

Nobody cares how unfit you are.

Nobody cares if you're not as fit as you were before.

The main thing people care about in a club when someone new joins is that you want to be a part of their community. They'll be delighted that you've decided to take the plunge, get back into your sport and make positive changes to your life.

TAKE-HOME HABIT

If this idea is striking a chord, put the book down right now, get online and find your local team, see when they practise and put it in your diary. You can thank me later.

37. RECONFIGURE YOUR KITCHEN

Is your kitchen an 'obesogenic environment'? That means it's *'an environment that promotes gaining weight and one that is not conducive to weight loss'.*[67]

If the answer is yes, don't worry.

There are some simple things that have been discovered by researchers at Cornell University, New York,[68] that you can do to re-engineer the kitchen to transform it from a place of weight-loss misery to fat loss mastery.

Fill the fruit bowl

Simply filling a fruit bowl with at least two types of fruit and placing it within 2 feet of the kitchen door can increase your fruit intake by 104%! It comes down to the convenience factor: if it's accessible and ready to go, then you're more likely to grab an apple or an orange than rummaging in the fridge or behind closed cupboard doors. Another tip for upping your fruit intake is to prepare snack-sized tubs and keep them handy in the fridge. Chop up some melon, pineapple or mango, or make a berry fruit salad – you know, the tasty fruits that we hardly ever eat because we can't be bothered to do the prep? Make some fruit pots when you're doing your weekly meal prep and it will also save you a few quid if you usually just buy these ready-prepared packs on the go.

Cut the clutter

The same researchers found that messy kitchens can lead to out-of-control eating. They found that participants with newspapers, bills, phones, tubs, packets and other clutter lying around on the worktops ate double the number of biscuits and snacks compared with those who had clearer counter-tops.

Keep the veg on top

Most fridges have a compartment at the bottom for storing fruits and veg, but the researchers found that if you flip the fridge layout and keep the fruits on top and the less healthy foods in the drawer, you'll eat 3 times as much just because it's more visible.

Serve from the kitchen

When bowls of food were placed on the table and folk were allowed the freedom to serve themselves, they ate 20% more than when the food was served from the kitchen onto individual plates. When you're free-serving you're far more likely to eat more than you actually need and it's much harder to remember what you're eating. This is especially problematic if you're keeping a food diary or tracking calories.

TAKE-HOME HABIT

You can turn your kitchen into a 'fat-fighting environment' by making some simple tweaks like giving the surfaces a good de-cluttering and keeping a full and varied fruit bowl in plain sight.

38. BE REALISTIC ABOUT YOUR DAILY CALORIES

'I'm only eating 1,000 calories and I'm not losing weight...'
I hate to break it to you, but you're not eating 1,000 calories.

» Here's why

As we talked about in the beginning, your body will not hold onto fat if you create a calorie deficit; it will burn it as needed for fuel until its need for energy is balanced. If you have a calorie requirement of 2,000 kcals per day (remember this is always an estimation and a moving target) and eat 2,000 kcals per day, you should maintain weight. If you consistently ate 3,000 kcals, you'd gain weight. If you ate 1,500 kcals, you'd lose weight.

When you factor in the calories burned in your daily activities, your metabolic rate, the energy your body uses to digest food, the calories you burn in exercise, your NEAT levels, and so on, when they are all added together it's extremely unlikely that a healthy adult could maintain their weight on 1,000 calories per day!

So what's happening?

Well, what this means is that you're probably, through no fault of your own, underestimating your intake.

Don't worry – we all do this. One study showed 25% of participants thought their meals had 500 fewer calories than they actually had.[69] Another study in obese people who reported a low-calorie intake showed some under-reported by up to 2,000 calories a day.[70] Even dietitians have been found to under-report their intake![71]

But don't worry. The good thing is that this is quite easy to fix.

Often you just need to shake things up a bit and try some new habits that will help you to burn more calories, eat fewer calories or simply become more mindful of what you're actually eating.

You just need to 'audit' your tracking and be super-honest and accurate.

» Log everything
Your breakfast, snacks, protein shakes, fancy coffees, fruit, everything you eat, in order to get the most from it if you actually want to make real progress. Don't skip meals and don't lie to yourself. Scan barcodes, use food scales, don't just eye-ball food portions.

Do this for a few days and you'll get a much clearer idea of what you're actually eating.

TAKE-HOME HABIT

Underestimating our calorie intake is very common and easy to do. When you're logging your food – on an app or in a diary – make sure you're accurate to get the most from it.

39. DOWNSIZE THE PLATE TO DROP THE WEIGHT

Eating your main meal off a smaller plate is a simple bit of kitchen re-engineering that can help reduce your calorie intake by up to 30%.[72] Researchers at Cornell University reported that when diners reduced their plate diameter by 30% (moving from a 12-inch dinner plate to a 9-inch plate), they ate 30% fewer calories as a result.

This happens for two reasons

- Firstly, and the most obvious reason: there is simply less room on the plate to pile on the potatoes, pasta and pakora.

- Secondly, and this is where it gets quite interesting, is that we become victims of the Delboeuf Illusion.[73] Our mind is tricked. Because the plate looks full, our mind and, in turn, our stomach believe that we are actually eating a lot more food.

Look at the image below: the amount of food on the plate on the right looks bigger than on the plate on the left, when in fact it's the same size.

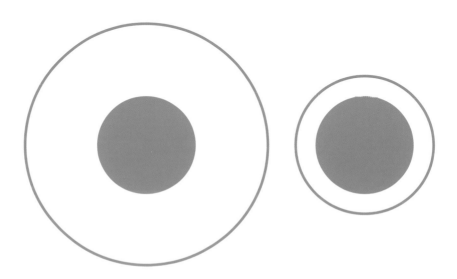

The smaller plate tactic is one of those fat-loss tools that everyone thinks they won't fall for, but we all do.

Harnessing the Delboeuf Illusion works regardless of what you're serving. If eating something in a bowl, get a smaller one; if you're having a drink, use a smaller glass. Whether you're going for some cereal or carbonara, pick the smaller plate!

TAKE-HOME HABIT

Switch to a smaller plate and you'll end up eating fewer calories. If you have a buffet lunch in the canteen, then this habit is one that you should definitely think about starting ASAP.

40. STEER CLEAR OF MEDIA SCAREMONGERING

If you want confusing, sensationalised, 'fake nutrition news' supported by very little evidence, read the newspapers.

Here's a classic example of two tabloid headlines:

'Yes, you CAN eat carbs! Expert reveals the 5 best recipes to keep you slim and full of energy – and stop you getting 'hangry'.[74]

'Cut carbs, quit sugar, feel fabulous: It's a food revolution that'll make you slimmer and happier – and it's blissfully simple.[75]

Confused? I would be.

If you read something about nutrition in the papers then you should take it with a pinch of salt. A 2012 study found that 72% of health claims made by newspapers were misleading.[76] Oh dear.

The problem is that moderation doesn't sell. Writing an article about balance or eating plenty of fruit and vegetables is not sexy.

Talking about 'superfoods' or secret fat-burning supplements that you must buy or the hidden toxic dangers of kale or some other garbage, unfortunately, does.

Another problem with newspaper reporting is that journalists love to muddy the water between correlations and causations, as explained in Cure Cravings with Diet Drinks (page 16).

» Here are a few simple tips for how you can level-up your bullsh*t detector

- If something sounds too good to be true, it probably is.

- If a single food is reported to significantly increase/decrease life expectancy, the chances are it's garbage.

- If only one study has been referenced, don't set too much store by it.

- If the study was done on animals, be wary – the findings don't always apply to humans.

- If any food or supplement is described as 'fat-burning', stop reading.

TAKE-HOME HABIT

Don't make any drastic changes to your lifestyle based on stories you've read in the newspapers. Try to remain critical and avoid snap decisions.

41. TURN OFF THE TV & DINE AT THE TABLE

Did you know that families who frequently eat dinner in the kitchen or dining room have significantly lower BMIs for both adults and children compared with families who eat elsewhere?[77]

It seems TV is to blame, again, for making us overweight.[78] **When we're distracted, we eat more. Research has shown that we indulge in more calories if we read and eat, use the computer on our lunch break, watch TV or even listen to music.**[79]

The type of TV programme you watch can also impact how much you eat. Unsurprisingly, watching food-related TV programmes impacts our eating behaviour.[80] Our level of interest also has an impact.

If we're interested in the programme, we eat more because we're thinking more about if Sheila is going to discover that Jimmy is having an affair with Betty next door, rather than how much we've eaten.[81]

Watching TV while eating also exposes you to the adverts. Studies have shown that food advertising increases our food consumption. The scary thing is that it's not just for the foods we see advertised, it simply increases our food intake overall![82]

My rule is generally to avoid buying food if you've seen it on TV.

Have you seen the advert of a super-hot model walking down a beach stroking a head of broccoli? No, of course you haven't. Broccoli – or any vegetables for that matter – isn't sexy food. But you will have seen the same advert where the model was seductively eating a calorie-laden tub of ice cream or type of chocolate-loaded biscuit.

TAKE-HOME HABIT

If you want to lose weight, don't watch TV while you eat, and if you want to improve the waistline of the entire family, make it a rule that all meals must be eaten at the dinner table.

42. STOP STRESSING OVER SCALE WEIGHT

The scale can be your friend.
'Yay! I lost 2lb!'

Or it can be your foe.
'I've gained a pound since last night.'

Sound familiar?

Here's the truth. Unless you're a boxer, jockey, weightlifter or you compete in a weight-restricted sport, it doesn't matter what weight you are.

Let that sink in for a minute.

The reason you're reading this book isn't because you want to lose *insert your weight loss goal here*. You might think it is, but trust me, it isn't. It's just a number. You're reading this book because you want to experience the positive emotions that you expect will come because of the weight loss. It's not really about a number at all; it's about feelings.

» Another thing

Your scale weight will fluctuate all over the place based on factors like your stomach content, hormones, hydration, toilet routine and many other factors, that are sometimes out of your control.

Therefore, what the scale tells you shouldn't be the be-all and end-all. Sure, it is ONE of the tools that you can use to track your progress. Losing 1 to 2 lb or 0.5 to 1kg a week seems to be a healthy target that is both realistic, and helps to minimise rebounds.[83]

However, it shouldn't be the only tool you use.

Progress photos are a great tool. Once you've read this book, go ahead and take three – one from the front, one from the side and one from the back. Take the same photos every month in the same place and use them to see and chart your changes.

Get a tape measure and, as a minimum, measure yourself around your stomach and hips. As with the photos, re-measure every month.

You can also track your progress based on how clothes feel – if your belt is a little looser or your shirt isn't so tight around your neck, this is progress too.

To download a progress tracking tool, head over to weightlossbook.co.uk/resources

TAKE-HOME HABIT

They say that if you want to progress in something, you need to track it. For fat loss, this needn't be scale weight. A combo of weight, photos and measurements is going to be less frustrating and more motivating in the long run.

43. REMEMBER: NOBODY LIKES A CHEATER

Cheat on your spouse; you'll end up single. Cheat in sport and you won't get to play again. Cheat your mates when playing FIFA and... you get the idea. None of the outcomes are good. The same goes for 'cheating on your diet'.

Note: Cheat meals are not the same as a 'refeed meal'. See Refuel with a Refeed Day (page 54) for more.

First, let's clarify the 'cheat meal'. Proponents claim that a weekly cheat meal is a great way to 'trick your body' and to 'rev up your metabolism' and that it's the key to getting lean. It's not.

» Here's the problem

Your weekly calorie deficit can be completely wiped out by a cheat meal. Look at it this way, let's say you're in a nice 15–20% per day calorie deficit. Hypothetically, let's say that's 300 calories per day. Over 6 days that would be a reduction of 1,800 calories, great. On the 7th day you include a cheat meal: a whole pizza, a couple of beers and some ice cream. Not only can that wipe out your deficit, but it could also move you into a calorie surplus, thereby increasing your weight. Not good.

'But Scott, my favourite Instagrammer is shredded and they love their weekly cheat meal...'

If you ate nothing but tofu and broth 9 times a day you'd be the same! Come the weekend they're so bored of their terrible diet that they're gagging for some form of flavour.

You are not them.

Moderation is the key here. Rather than going into full-on restriction mode during the week, make sure you include foods that you actually like.

80% of your calories should be nutritious, whole foods, with 20% leeway for less nutritious, but extremely tasty foods you love.

This will keep you sane.

This will help you get lean.

This will stop you ruining your progress with a cheat meal at the weekend because your mid-week food is so boring!

TAKE-HOME HABIT

Cheaters never win. Make sure you structure your mid-week eating so that you actually enjoy it and it's not extremely restrictive, forcing you into 'cheating' at the weekend!

44. GET OUTSIDE TO WORK OUT

As a kid you were probably fed up with being told to get off the sofa, turn off the TV and get outside. Well, Mum was onto something, you know. There are quite a few benefits to exercising outdoors that you don't get in a gym.

» **You can burn more calories exercising outside**
Researchers at the University of Exeter found that if you're a runner, you'll burn more calories outside compared with running on a treadmill.[84] This is because of wind resistance, which makes you work harder.

» **Exercise releases endorphins (feel-good hormones)**
So does spending more time in 'green spaces'.[85] So if you combine the two and exercise outdoors then you're on to a winner. It can improve your mood and reduce depression.[86]

» **You'll get a much-needed hit of vitamin D**
Apparently 50% of the population are deficient in the sunshine vitamin.[87] Vitamin D reduces the risk of many chronic diseases e.g. autoimmune diseases, type 2 diabetes, heart disease, and many cancers and infectious diseases. And it can boost your self-esteem.[88]

» **It's cheap – you don't need a gym membership.**
(Why would someone pay for a gym membership to use a treadmill?!)

» **It's accessible**
Open your front door and boom! You're at the outdoor playground already.

TAKE-HOME HABIT

If you can work out outside, go for it. Instead of doing your HIIT workout inside, go to the garden. Take a kettlebell to the park. Run up a hill, not on a treadmill, and reap the benefits of outdoor exercise.

45. 'NO PAIN, NO GAIN' IS FOR NUMPTIES

The no-pain, no-gain mentality that worked for Rocky Balboa coupled with the copious memes you will have seen about the 'feeling after leg day' might make you think that exercise is a waste of time unless you struggle to walk by the end. Having DOMS (Delayed Onset Muscle Soreness) – that sore feeling after a tough workout – is a futile high that many chase each and every time they head to the gym or go for a run.

» Here's the deal

DOMS is caused by connective tissue and muscle damage.[89] This causes inflammation, hence the discomfort. It is most likely experienced after a new training stimulus (a change to exercises or volume), not simply after a 'hardcore workout'.

If you're using exercise alongside diet to burn fat, then your primary goals are to burn as many calories in the workout as possible and to maintain muscle mass (see Build Muscle to Burn Fat on page 114). Your goal is not to brutalise your body so that it takes days for you to recover, increase your risk of injury or force yourself through a type of workout that you hate.

Although high-intensity workouts have a lot of benefits,[90] they also have relatively poor adherence[91] and, as you should know by now, adherence is key. The goal of this book is to give you a load of ideas that will help you to lose weight, and I want you to pick the ones that you'll enjoy and stick with.

If high-intensity workouts aren't for you, don't do them!

TAKE-HOME HABIT

A workout should be appropriate for your goals and abilities. Despite what you'll see on Instagram, it doesn't need to be 'brutal' and 'hardcore,' and adherence is the number one factor. Do what you enjoy!

46. EMBRACE INTUITIVE EATING & DITCH DIETS

Intuitive eating is an anti-diet concept that is growing in popularity. Perhaps its success is because it offers an alternative to the 'clean eating' culture, provides a respite for perpetual dieters and partly because it just makes sense.

The term 'Intuitive Eating' was first coined by Evelyn Tribole and Elyse Resch in their 1995 book of the same name.[92] There isn't a lot of research on the topic, but the studies that have been done show it improves our attitude towards food, lowers BMI and helps with weight maintenance.[93]

Here are the 10 principles covered in the book:

1. Reject the Diet Mentality
Stop looking for the next quick fix and flip-flopping between diets. If you've tried countless diets in the past, and they've never worked, that should be reason enough to stop searching for the next quick fix.

2. Honor Your Hunger
Don't starve yourself. If you're hungry, eat. Going hungry for lengthy periods is just likely to make you overeat when you do finally stop restricting your biological desire for food.

3. Make Peace with Food
Stop the food fights. Don't unnecessarily restrict and deprive yourself of any foods. When you do finally break your self-imposed restriction, you're likely to binge because of your prolonged deprivation.

4. Challenge the Food Police
Food isn't 'good' or 'bad', it's not 'clean' or 'dirty'. Food is food and it doesn't need a label.

5. Respect Your Fullness
Listen to your body. Eat what you need but don't go overboard, stop when you're no longer hungry yet you feel satisfied.

6. Discover the Satisfaction Factor
Food is a wonderful thing and it should be enjoyed, not feared or unnecessarily restricted. Eat in a friendly, happy environment, savour the food, the company and the people you share it with.

7. Honor Your Feelings Without Using Food
Don't use food as your cure for a bad day, an argument or any other negative feelings. Food won't solve the problem and emotional eating will only make it worse in the long run.

8. Respect Your Body
Appreciate your figure and who you are, don't be overly critical about your body size or shape.

9. Exercise – Feel the Difference
Move more. It doesn't have to be hard exercise (like I've been saying) simply get moving and be active.

10. Honor Your Health
You don't need a perfect diet. One snack or meal isn't going to make the slightest difference; it's a long-term game.

TAKE-HOME HABIT

The easiest way to start with intuitive eating is to become more mindful of what you eat, when you eat and how it makes you feel.

47. EAT THAT FROG & WORK OUT FIRST THING

I'm not sure what the protein content of a frog is, but before you get all grossed-out I am not actually suggesting you start munching on some web-footed amphibians for your breakfast.

'Eat That Frog' is a concept popularised by success coach Brian Tracy.[94] His book is based on the idea that if the worst thing you must do in a day is to eat a frog, do it first and get it over and done with. If exercise is your 'frog', get it done and dusted as soon as you can.

You'll be able to get more enjoyment from the rest of your day without it looming over your head and, secondly, you'll experience that satisfied and accomplished after-exercise-feeling for the entire day.

From a physiological standpoint, there doesn't seem to be an advantage to exercising in the morning compared with later in the day. Morning exercise may slightly supress your appetite more than evening exercise, which could be a good thing.[95] However, for both cardiovascular and resistance training, it doesn't seem to matter what time of day you exercise.[96] The outcomes will be largely the same. When you train should be down to your own preference, schedule, energy levels and so on. So, if you find that you're one of those people who say 'I don't mind it once I get there, it's having the motivation to go...' then getting your exercise done first thing is probably a smart move.

Let's say you decide to work out first thing, you might have heard that exercising on an empty stomach is better for fat loss? The theory is that your body will burn more body fat if you haven't eaten anything. However, the research[97] shows us that it doesn't matter if you decide to eat beforehand or not, the results will be the same.

While there might not be a strong physiological reason for exercising in the morning, there are several psychological reasons why it might be a good thing.

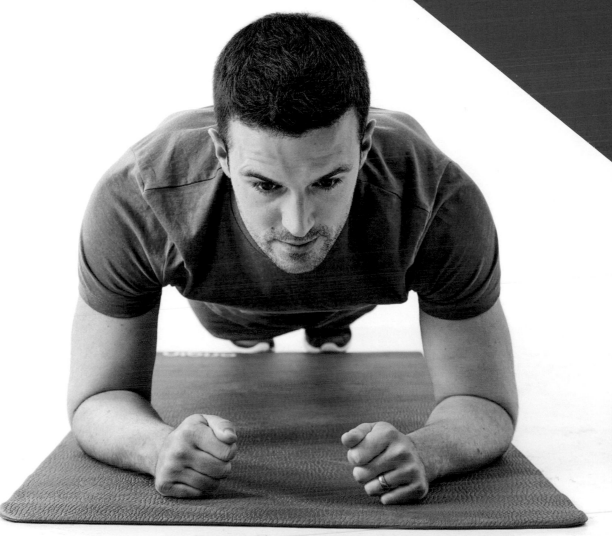

48. PRIORITISE PROGRESSIVE OVERLOAD

'*The definition of insanity is doing the same thing over and over again and expecting a different result.*' This is often attributed to Albert Einstein, but did you know there isn't any evidence that he wrote or spoke that statement?[98]

Anyway, I digress. The point is, if you do the same thing over and over again in the gym you're not going to see any progress.

If you lift weights, you need to embrace the most important rule of strength training – progressive overload.[99]

You will only get stronger if you constantly increase the demands on your muscles. If you always pick your favourite exercises, do the same reps for the same number of sets then you're going to be perpetually stuck in NoGainsville.

Even if you're not trying to become the next Arnie, you don't want to get complacent with your training.

Here are some of the ways of putting progressive overload into practice:

>> **Increase the weight**
This is probably the easiest option. You don't need to go lifting the heavier dumbbells every time you hit the gym or slamming new plates onto the bar for every lift, but you do need to track how much you're lifting and gradually increase this over time.

>> **Up the reps**
If you always do 10 squats, 10 dumbbell curls and 10 lunges, simply doing 11 is a form of progressive overload.

» Lift the same weight but with better form and increase control

You want to become a master of technique. If your technique is poor, then you're not going to be as efficient with your energy as you could be. By improving your form, you'll be able to lift the same weight with less energy, which means you'll be more likely to increase the weight over time.

» Increase the volume

You could add in an extra set or perhaps an extra exercise.

» Reduce rest periods and training time

If you do the same amount of work and lift the same volume but in less time, that is a form of progressive overload.

» Lift more often

Increase your training frequency. If you train once a week, add in another session.

TAKE-HOME HABIT

Don't just wing it when you go to the gym. Take a note of what you lift and how much you lift so that over time you can implement a form of progressive overload so you don't plateau.

49. FOCUS ON THE PROCESS, NOT THE OUTCOME

When it comes to goal-setting, as tempting as it may be, you want to focus more on the process and not the outcome.

» Here's what I mean

An outcome goal might be to lose 15kg. When you have an outcome goal it can become an obsessive target. It ends up controlling you. This arbitrary weight on the scale can consume you and if you lose less one week than you did the week before you'll feel deflated. If you lose 14.9kg, you don't care – it's not the 15 that you wanted.

Outcome goals can also push you adopt extreme, unpleasant habits that aren't sustainable and didn't work for you in the past. Juice detox, anyone? Whatever it takes.

You also don't really have that much control over an outcome goal. Sure, you can do things that will help you lose weight but if, and how much weight you actually lose, is down to your body, it's not up to you.

Here's the deal: when you focus on the process, you have control; you're in charge.

With process goals, you stop seeing weight loss as a means to an end.[100] You focus on actions, behaviours and choices that, if practised over time, will lead to the outcome goal. For example, process goals would be committing to follow pretty much any habit in this book: include protein at breakfast, do 10,000 steps each day, eat dinner at the table, work out first thing in the morning, etc.

'I will persist until I succeed. Always will I take another step. If that is of no avail I will take another, and yet another. In truth, one step at a time is not too difficult… I know that small attempts, repeated, will complete any undertaking.'
Og Mandino

Another thing to reiterate that I mentioned in Stop Stressing over Scale Weight (page 96), is that scale weight fluctuates, and it can be frustrating and disheartening when it's the only goal you're focusing on. By practising small, daily habits and by focusing on the process, you'll avoid the highs and lows of 'Woo-hoo! I lost a pound' and 'FML, I gained a pound'.

TAKE-HOME HABIT

Focus on the process and concentrate on developing behaviours and habits instead of fixating on the outcome. This is easier to do, more fulfilling, less stressful and will result in lasting weight-loss success.

50. LIMIT YOUR LIQUID CALORIES

One of the easiest weight-loss habits that you could adopt would be to avoid liquid calories.

You don't need science to tell you that sugary, calorie-laden drinks aren't great if you're trying to lose weight.[101]

The problem with liquid calories is that in most cases they're very un-satiating because there isn't any fibre or protein. Your digestive system also doesn't have to do much work in order to extract the energy from drinks because they're already easily digestible, with no bulk to break down in the first place.

Aside from the simple switch of changing a regular fizzy drink for a diet version, as we discuss in Cure Cravings with Diet Drinks (page 16), or rethinking your coffees (Change up Your Coffees on page 44), or being aware of calorific alcohol (Keep Tabs on Your Bar Tab on page 150), there are a few other occasions when liquid calories may cross your path. When I see people in the gym doing some cardio to help them lose weight, my heart breaks a little if I see them swigging on a sports drink at the same time.

Burn 150 calories on a treadmill.
Drink 150 calories from a sports drink.
Change in calories: 0. Weight loss: 0.

If you're exercising for less than an hour, you don't need to have any form of carbohydrate during a workout. You only need to be thinking about topping up your carbohydrate reserves if you're doing some form of cardio that lasts longer than an hour. For anything less than that, water will be just fine. If you need some flavour, add some no-sugar squash or buy the 'zero' variety of sports drink instead.

Another time liquid calories appear in the diet is when people hear that smoothies and juicing are good ideas and throw half an orchard into a blender.

Smoothies can be a smart move if you need something that's easily digestible before a workout in the morning (see Pile on the Protein at Breakfast on page 20), but other than that I'd avoid them.

Yes, you can add in fruits and veg and other 'healthy' foods and benefit from the vitamins contained within, but it's very easy to go overboard and you're less likely to overeat whole foods compared with liquidised foods.

TAKE-HOME HABIT

To drastically reduce your overall calorie intake (depending on how much you drink at the moment), cut back on liquid calories and find a lower-calorie or calorie-free alternative.

51. GET MORE KIP TO MOVE MORE KILOS

You already know that sleep is important. I'm not going to harp on about something you know already. However, did you know that a lack of sleep has been shown to interfere with your fat-loss efforts?

For starters, folk who regularly get fewer than 6 hours' sleep per night have a higher BMI compared to those who get a longer night's kip[102]. Sleeping for fewer than 6 hours also decreases leptin (a hormone which helps to keep you feeling full) and increases ghrelin (a hormone that makes you feel hungry)![103]

It continues... A study in *The American Journal Of Clinical Nutrition* found that when people were sleep-deprived, they scoffed more snacks in the evening and ate around an extra 200 calories.[104]

From an exercise perspective, sleep is a key element to helping you recover, replenish and rebuild. Secondly, if you're frequently sleep-deprived, your exercise performance isn't gong to be as good as it could be either.[105]

Getting more sleep could be a really simple habit to implement. All you need to do is commit to switching off the video game, putting down the magazine and powering down the TV by a set time.

Even if you get an extra 30 minutes, it's an improvement.

Here are some other tips to get a better kip:

» **Set yourself a bedtime**
I know you're not 7 years old, but pick a time to go to bed during the week and stick to it. Try to have a regular routine and go to bed around the same time and wake at the same time each morning.

» **You can catch up on sleep at the weekend**
But don't go overboard to the extent that you can't fall asleep at your usual bedtime.

» **Avoid using devices that emit blue light, like phones and tablets, before you go to sleep**
These have been shown to disrupt your circadian rhythm and make it harder to wander in the land of nod.[106]

» **Don't get your mind excited before sleeping**
Try to read some fiction that will help you to relax rather than reading something like a book for work which is likely to be filled with numbers, facts and important things you should remember.

» **Practise some relaxation techniques before bed**
There are lots of free meditation or yoga apps that will help to quieten your mind before lights-out time.

TAKE-HOME HABIT

If you get fewer than 6 hours per night, set a sleep goal and go to bed earlier. It's a simple habit that could have serious results.

52. BUILD MUSCLE TO BURN FAT

Wait, I thought this was a book about losing weight and burning fat, not building muscle?

Well, did you know that if you've got more muscle, you'll burn more fat?

Muscle tissue is metabolically active; it uses more calories than body fat does. Generally, the more muscle you have, the higher your basal metabolic rate will be (this is the number of calories your body burns when you're at rest). Let's say you're 80kg with 30% body fat. That means that of your 80kg, 24kg is fat, so your lean body mass is 56kg. If you were 80kg but only 10% body fat, only 8kg is fat, so your lean body mass is 72kg. More muscle = more calories being burned.

So, how do you build muscle?

Make sure you eat enough protein
You'll know by now that protein is important for a host of functions from helping to keep you feeling full to repairing muscle tissue. Some studies[107] suggest that 1.6–1.8g of protein per kg of bodyweight would be a sensible target to aim for if muscle gain is the goal. Think plenty of chicken, fish, turkey, beans and pulses, dairy and eggs.

Eat enough calories
This will seem counterintuitive to everything else in the book. I get it. Unfortunately, it's very hard to build muscle when you're in a calorie deficit (what we've been striving for this entire book). You need to go past maintenance calories (when your calories in matches calories out) and move into a calorie surplus (when you consume more calories than you burn per day). You can be smart and cycle your calories and achieve the elusive goal of body re-composition (when you build muscle and burn fat at the same time). To do this you would typically eat around 10% more calories than your maintenance on days when you lift weights, and stick to your calorie deficit on rest days.

Get stronger

Focus on the big lifts in a reasonably low rep range. This means deadlifts, squats, lunges and pressing at around 85–90% of your 1 rep max, which will generally mean your reps will be in the 3–7 range.[108]

Take creatine monohydrate

If your goals are to increase muscle size, improve power output and get stronger, then supplementing with creatine is probably going to help. A meta-analysis in the *Journal of Strength & Conditioning Research*[109] reviewed 22 studies on creatine and weightlifting performance and found creatine increased strength by 8% and power output by 14%. Another study[110] reviewed 100 papers on creatine and showed that creatine was proven to increase muscle mass.

TAKE-HOME HABIT

If you don't have very much muscle on your frame at the moment, set a goal to build more if you want to burn more fat.

53. MAKE SOME RULES; SET UP A SYSTEM

As soon as you've decided on your 30-day SMART goals, you need to create systems to make it happen.

What's the difference between a goal and a system?

New York Times bestselling author Scott Adams says:
'*A goal is a specific objective that you either achieve or don't sometime in the future. A system is something you do on a regular basis that achieves your odds of happiness in the long run. If you do something every day, it's a system. If you're waiting to achieve it someday in the future, it's a goal.*'[111]

The goal is to lose weight. To achieve said goal you need to create a set of rules and systems that will help you to implement the habits in the book.

» For example

- You will lift weights for 30 minutes, at least 3 times a week.

- If you're going to be exercising you will have a coffee (see Chug a Coffee before a Workout on page 178) and eat a protein- and carb-rich meal both before and after training (Eat, Exercise, Repeat on page 146).

- Upon waking you will do 10 minutes of meditation each day (Meditate to Lose Weight on page 170).

- Every Sunday afternoon you will prep at least 2 different meals that make at least 4 portions each (Plan Ahead & Cook in Bulk on page 118).

- Before going to bed you will complete your daily journal (Jump into Journalling on page 140).

- If you're not exercising that day you will stand at your desk for at least 60 minutes (Stand More to Burn More on page 186).

- You will eat breakfast every day before you go to work (Pile on the Protein at Breakfast on page 20).

Systems can be triggered based on certain cues. Stephen Guise[112] talks about three different types of cues that trigger a habit.

Activity-based cues happen based on events that occur every day. For example, when you get to work you'll take the stairs not the lift; when you get to the gym you'll do 10 minutes of cardio after a weights workout; when you get home you'll have a glass of water, before you go to bed you'll write your journal.

Time-based cues are habits that are triggered at set times throughout the day. For example, at 11AM you'll have a snack, at 7PM you'll eat dinner, at 9PM you'll go to bed.

Flexible daily cues can be done whenever you like so long as you've completed them before you go to bed.

'Success is the sum of small habits repeated day in and day out.' R. Collier

My goal was to write this book. My system was to write 3 'ways' every day as soon as I turned on the computer, before I did any other jobs, before I checked email or scrolled through social media. It was hard at first; I wanted to look on Facebook to see what was happening but after a week it became the norm. Computer on, chapters written. It works.

You're reading the result of having a solid system in place.

TAKE-HOME HABIT

If you've got systems in place, it makes the achievement of the goal much quicker. It removes the decision-making process, becomes the norm and allows you to focus on other areas. It becomes an automated process: if you do X then you do Y.

54. PLAN AHEAD & COOK IN BULK

I interviewed fat-loss coach Josh Hillis on 'The Food For Fitness Podcast' and one of my favourite things that he said was that meal prep was the most important workout of the week.

I love that – it's an expression I'll always use.

He's so right. Meal prep is one workout that you need to schedule into your plan and that you've got to keep. Failure to prepare is preparing to fail.

We can go all day with these – here's another. An old teacher of mine always talked about the 7 Ps: Proper Prior Planning Prevents P*** Poor Performance.

You get the idea.

But guess what? There are even studies that show meal prep decreases your chances of being overweight.[113]

Are you someone who comes home from work and just can't be bothered to cook and ends up grabbing something quick and calorie-laden? Perhaps you're prone to ordering a mid-week takeaway or you just eat a load of snack foods in the cupboard because it's easy. If so, you've got to start meal prepping.

» Here's how you do it

Set some time aside on a Sunday afternoon, get some tunes on or set up your tablet in the kitchen with a film on and get to it.

Stews, casseroles, curries, one-pot dishes. Go to town. Don't waste time on cooking meals that serve 1 or 2. Cook like you're cooking for 6. Divide the dish into individual portions and freeze some of them. That will give you plenty of dinners and options to take in for lunch the next day too.

A slow cooker is also a winner if you're pressed for time (see Get into Slow Cooking on page 34). You whack all of the ingredients into it before you go to work, set it to cook for 8 hours on low and when you get in at 5 you're greeted with amazing food smells and a delicious pot of food waiting for you in the kitchen. If you don't have one, get one!

When I cook, it's extremely rare that I'll cook a meal that does fewer than 4 portions.

Why? Because as much as I love cooking, I can't be bothered to cook every night of the week – not unlike a lot of people!

TAKE-HOME HABIT

Schedule some time into your calendar to cook up some big pots of food for the week and beyond so you've always got a healthy option in the fridge or freezer if you're pressed for time.

55. REWARD YOURSELF & HIT THOSE TARGETS

Sometimes we need a little extra help.

It's a cold, dark and 'dreich' (as we say in Scotland) winter's morning and the thought of climbing out of your cosy bed and heading off to the gym is as appealing as sharing your protein shaker with someone who has norovirus.

Incentivising is one of my favourite tools for helping folk lose weight.

Surely by this point, you will have nailed down some 30-day SMART goals. If not, you need to read Make a Plan, Not Just a Wish (page 38). Once you've got your goals cemented, you need to pick non-food rewards if you hit them. This means that you don't celebrate with a huge night out on the lash and undo all of your hard work.

Let's say you're aiming to lose 0.5–1kg a week, every week for a month. If you hit the lower goal then you get one reward, if you hit the higher one you get another.

Rewards that help you hit the next target are going to be even better. For example, you could get new pair of trainers, a massage, new headphones, a PT session, some home gym equipment and so on.

You could also buy that amazing new dress or swag shirt you've had your eyes on. The catch is you have to buy it a size smaller than you can fit into at the moment... And throw away the receipt, too.

If you've got kids, I love to encourage people to get them involved, too.

If you hit your target for the month, let them know that you'll take them to for a day out or that they'll get a reward too. They'll keep you accountable – probably more than you would like but this is going to be for the greater good.

If you've got your habit tracker up on the fridge door, let them do the box-ticking or gold star-pinning for you. If you've not printed yours yet, make sure to get it from the resources area at weightlossbook.co.uk.

TAKE-HOME HABIT

Set rewards if you hit your target and if you want to get some added accountability, reward family and loved ones too.

56. GET A BOOST WITH THE MASTER BLASTER

Joe Weider was a bit of a legend in fitness and bodybuilding circles. Known as 'The Master Blaster', he created the International Federation of Bodybuilders (IFBB) and many of the most popular fitness mags like *Muscle & Fitness*, *Shape* and *Men's Fitness*.

He also popularised several weight-lifting techniques which became known as the Weider Principles.[114] Now, I'll be the first to admit that some of them are perhaps a bit 'old school bodybuilding-esque' but there are several, which we'll focus on, that will help take your weights training up a level.

Muscle Priority principle

Weider suggested that you focus on your weakest body part first in the workout when your energy levels are highest. I suggest doing your least favourite exercises first, and 'eat that frog', as we discussed on page 104. Basically, get the hardest, least enjoyable exercises done first and save the best until last.

Holistic Training principle

This approach recommends that you don't always pick the same exercises and do the same reps in the same order. Weider recommended that followers change up the rep ranges. For example, if you always do 6–8 reps for a given exercise try 12–15 or 15–20 instead. He also recommended that you change exercise order and rep tempo, too. Don't just do the same thing over and over again.

Rest-Pause principle

On the final set of an exercise, once you've hit your rep target, take a short rest of up to 30 seconds then try and do a couple of extra reps. This is really going to push you past your comfort zone, which is why it's not a good idea to do it on every set of every exercise, just save it for the finishers.

Drop sets

Another technique to increase the intensity of a workout. Weider recommended that after you'd completed a set of an exercise, you immediately drop the weight and try and do another set, followed by a third.

Instinctive training

Listen to your body. If you go into the gym and you're still feeling sore from the last workout, this Weider principle says that you should adapt your programme accordingly: change the focus, do some cardio instead, use lighter weights. Just as we talked about on page 101 the 'no pain, no gain' mentality is only for idiots.

TAKE-HOME HABIT

A smart use of the Weider principles is a way that can help you to take your workouts from bro to pro.

57. CUT BACK; DON'T CUT OUT

When people start trying to improve the way they eat, they fixate on the things they think they can't eat. Their entire healthy eating regime is focused on exclusion.

No more chocolate for 30 days. Dry January. See you, sugar. Cut the carbs.

Sound familiar?

The only thing you should exclude from your diet is unnecessary exclusion. You don't need to stop eating bread unless it makes you ill. You don't need to stop eating chocolate unless it makes you ill. You don't need to stop eating sugar unless it makes you ill. See the trend here?

There are no foods or food groups that you must remove from your diet in order to lose fat.

I'll let that sink in for a moment.

The only time you need to remove something from your diet is if you don't like it or it makes you feel unwell when you eat it.

You will see so much garbage on social media and on bookshelves that blame a single food for the multifaceted obesity crisis. They tell you that sugar is poison, bread is destroying your gut and meat causes cancer. As a result, your first port of call when trying to eat better is usually to impose a ban on your favourite foods for an arbitrary length of time.

This doesn't work. If it did, you wouldn't be reading this book.

'So you're saying I can eat as much sugar as I like?'
No, I'm not.

What I am suggesting is that you think about ways to cut down on the foods that aren't really supporting your goals but don't remove them entirely. Going cold turkey will just make you feel deprived and you'll want to rebel against your unnecessarily restrictive your rule.

Go and read Embrace Intuitive Eating & Ditch Diets (page 102) for more about this.

Just try to cut back rather than cut out.

When making dietary changes, think of all the food you CAN eat. There are hundreds of varieties of fruit that you've probably never tasted; you probably buy the same vegetables and cook them exactly the same way week in, week out. You probably have 5–10 recipes you use and that's it. Get creative! Try something new!

TAKE-HOME HABIT

Don't impose unrealistic food bans on yourself and prioritise the positives – think what you can eat, not what you can't.

58. CHEW GUM TO CUT CARB CRAVINGS

Chewing gum can be a simple way to cut your cravings, unless you live in Singapore. (Chewing gum in the Asian city-state is actually illegal, so maybe skip this chapter if you're reading this book over there.[115])

Chewing on gum, especially in the afternoon, can boost your satiety score meaning that it tricks you into thinking you're fuller than you actually are.

One study in 50 overweight women found that those who had some gum between lunch and dinner snacked on less carb-heavy food in the afternoon compared with the group who didn't get any gum.[116] Another found similar results in men who hadn't eaten either.[117]

The mid-afternoon stomach rumbles can be a daily problem for many of us.

Aside from keeping some gum handy, here are a couple of other tips to defeat the hunger demons.

» **Add more protein to your lunch**
It also helps to keep you feeling full.

» **Put more fibre on your lunch plate**
Get more of those veggies in.

» Have a 'planned snack' break

Instead of just heading to the vending machine and grabbing something to satisfy your cravings, take some food from home with you to have between meals. Think fruit, yoghurts, a cereal bar, some jerky, a handful of nuts... Aim for something more filling and more nutritious than what you'd probably find in a vending machine.

» Have a cup of tea or a drink

Often we think we're hungry when, in fact, a drink will do us just fine for a while longer.

Be careful, though: it's been reported that some folk have unintentionally lost too much weight due to chewing too much gum. One study found that chewing too much gum led to a 20% loss in body weight due to chronic diarrhoea...[118] So let's not do anything silly, okay?

TAKE-HOME HABIT

Keep some chewing gum at the ready for combatting mid-afternoon carb cravings.

59. BLAST FAT WITH A BARBELL COMPLEX

Barbell complexes are the bee's knees.

A complex is usually a set of exercises, performed one after the other, with the same weight on the bar, with no rest between them. You only let go of the bar once you've finished all of the exercises.

Why are they so good? Well, for starters you're in and out of the gym in less time, you don't need to waste time changing the weight, they boost your heart rate and they're predominantly focused on compound movements (exercises that recruit a lot of muscle groups; more muscle groups = more calories burned).

Be warned: complexes are super-effective but they're tough. Remember that complexes are like HIIT cardio workouts (see Hop on the HIIT Bandwagon on page 22) – they're mainly going to challenge your cardiovascular system, not force you to shift as big a weight as possible. Only use the heaviest weight you can lift on your weakest lift in the series. Make sense?

Here are 4 of my favourites:

» **The Baptie Original**
This was the very first complex I did in the gym many moons ago and, to date, it's still one of my favourites. Perform 6 reps of each before letting the bar hit the floor: 6 x deadlifts, 6 x bent-over rows, 6 x power cleans, 6 x thrusters (front squat with an overhead press), then 6 x back squats.

» **Sumo Submission**
6 x sumo deadlifts, 6 x high pulls, 6 x front squats, 6 x overhead presses, then 6 x lunges.

» **Bear Complex – a favourite in CrossFit circles**
5 x power cleans, 5 x front squats, 5 x push presses, 5 x back squats, then 5 x push presses.

» **Romanian Rules**
5 x Romanian deadlifts, 5 x barbell rows, 5 x high pulls, 5 x push presses, then 5 x reverse lunges.

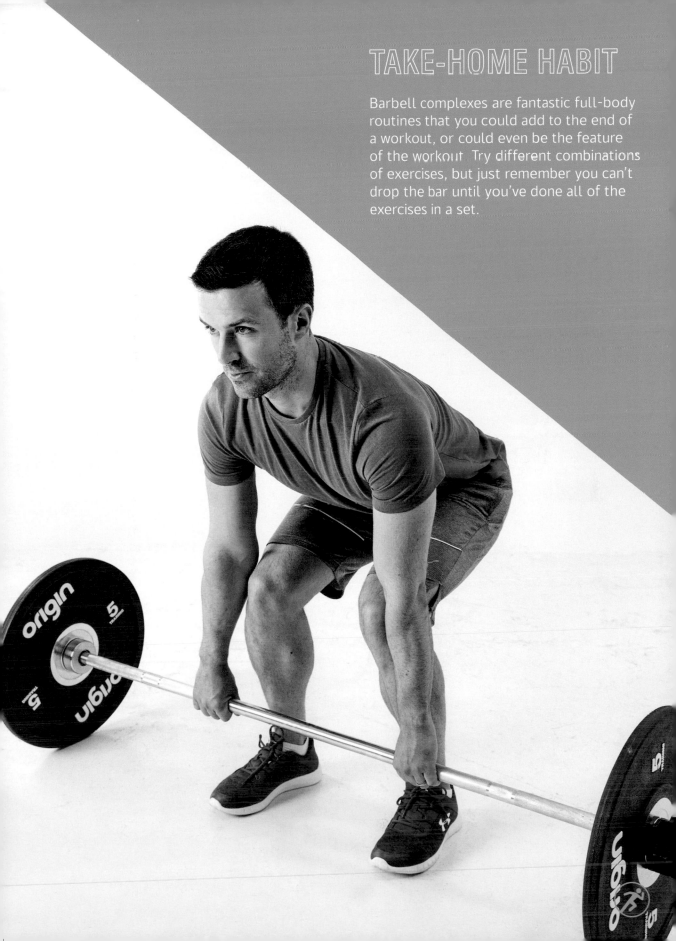

TAKE-HOME HABIT

Barbell complexes are fantastic full-body routines that you could add to the end of a workout, or could even be the feature of the workout. Try different combinations of exercises, but just remember you can't drop the bar until you've done all of the exercises in a set.

60. TREAT YOURSELF TO A DIET BREAK

'Diet break': two words that make you feel all warm and tingly, like when you find the scoop at the top of a new tub of protein.

If you've never heard of a diet break, well my friend, you're in for a treat.

It's a fairly simple concept but it can often be abused. The general idea is that if you've been in a calorie deficit, and you've been losing weight for around 12 weeks, you take some time off, typically for around a week.

When you take a diet break, you slightly increase your calories to around maintenance level, meaning your weight doesn't drop for the duration of the break.

The benefits are two-fold

- There is the psychological benefit in that some time off can be a huge boost. This is especially significant if you have a lot of weight to lose and the reality is that you'll need to be in a calorie deficit for months, if not years, to get to your ultimate goal weight.

- The physiological benefits of a break are that you'll feel less hungry, you'll have more energy, exercise performance will increase and certain hormones that are effected by weight loss get a chance to return to more normal levels.

The research also shows that diet breaks are more effective than continuous dieting. Nutritionists at the University of Tasmania found that participants who followed a 2:2 diet approach (2 weeks dieting, 2 weeks on a diet break) for 30 weeks lost more weight than the group who dieted continuously for the full duration.[119]

» How to implement a diet break

The most important thing to remember is that calories should be increased slightly to maintenance level. This means that you're eating about the same number of calories as you burn per day so your weight doesn't change. The mistake a lot of people make is that they think a diet break is a free-for-all and they go to excess and experience weight gain, just like when folk have cheat meals (see Remember: Nobody Likes a Cheater on page 98).

I'd suggest eating the same types of food, at roughly the same times as you would normally when you're losing weight, but just eat a little more at each meal, nothing crazy.

How often you want to take a break is down to you, but from working with my clients, I've found every 10 or 12 weeks seems to be the sweet spot.

TAKE-HOME HABIT

A planned and controlled diet break can be an excellent weapon in your fat-loss arsenal, if implemented intelligently and not used as an excuse to binge and erode all your hard work.

61. CONQUER THE SUPERMARKET

Most of us have experienced a strange phenomenon that occurs in shopping aisles across the land: sneaky foods just end up slinking into our trolleys.

We're not exactly sure how it happens but the most logical explanation is that when we turn our back to buy some broccoli and matcha, the chocolate bars jump into our trolley and bury themselves underneath the blueberries and spinach...

The weekly shopping trip can be the thing of nightmares, but here are some top tips to stop the supermarket sabotaging your progress.

Before you start the shop, make sure you don't go on an empty stomach. If we shop when we're hungry we buy more. One study found that participants who hadn't eaten in 5 hours prior to shopping bought more high-calorie foods than those who had a snack beforehand.[120]

Therefore, if you want to make the shop even better, one of the best pre-shopping snacks is an apple. Here's why: one study found that when the researchers gave shoppers an apple to eat before starting their shop, they bought 25% more fruit and veg.[121] Having a healthy snack primed the shoppers to buy healthier food.

Also, before you get to the shop, make sure you have a list. This ties into Plan Ahead & Cook in Bulk (page 118) when we spoke about meal prep being one of the most important workouts of the week. Once you've made your weekly food plan, head to the shops and only buy what you need and what's on your list. You'll cut down on food waste, eat a broader range of foods and you won't be tempted by all the buy-one-get-one-free offers for stuff you'll probably just chuck anyway.

Once you get to the shop, do most of your shopping on the outside aisles – that's where you'll find the fresh foods. Once you start to venture into the middle, you'll find nutrient density goes down and calorie load goes up.

Another tip is to divide your shopping trolley into two parts: one part is for fruit and veg, the other half for everything else. You can either do this in your head or use something like a jacket to create two compartments. When shoppers did this, researchers found that they bought more fruit and veg as a result.[122]

» Here's another idea

Why don't you scrap the trip to the supermarket completely and do your food shop online? It will save a load of time and, for a few quid (or free, in many cases), someone will do your shop for you and take it straight into your kitchen. One study found that online shopping decreased impulse buying and reduced the number of foods and high-fat snacks in the house.[123]

TAKE-HOME HABIT

Avoid going to the supermarket on an empty stomach. If you're hungry, grab an apple and, once you're there, split your trolley in two and do most of your shopping in the outside aisles.

62. MODERATE THE DRIED FRUIT INTAKE

I talked about why fruit is fantastic in Fight Fat with Fruit (page 80), but don't go tucking into your dried mango and sultanas mistakenly thinking they're the same as fruit. They're not.

Dried fruit has a hugely different nutritional profile to fresh fruit.

Here is the nutritional information for 100g of fresh mango:
Protein: 1g
Carbohydrates: 14g
Fat: 0g
Calories: 66

Compare that with 100g of dried mango:
Protein: 2g
Carbohydrates: 71g
Fat: 0g
Calories: 311

Pretty significant differences, right?

The water content is the kicker. Once it's removed, you've pretty much got an entirely different food in front of you. The sugar content significantly increases and it ramps up the calories 5-fold.

Although I've used mango as an example, this comparison pretty much applies to any fresh fruit and dried fruit. They're not the same. The macros and calories are extremely different!

Yes, the packaging might say 'counts as one of your five a day', but don't be fooled. I would pick the fresh fruit 99 times out of 100. It's more filling, you'll get the hydrating benefits of the water, and it contains a boat-load fewer calories.

Dried fruit can have its place.

Like any food, it's fine to eat, so long as you're aware of the energy value and the macros (no food is off limits, remember?).

If you're doing endurance sport for longer than an hour, dried fruit can be a great way to get a quick carb hit when you're out pounding the pavement or climbing a hill on your bike.

TAKE-HOME HABIT

No food is off limits, but I'd go for fresh fruit over dried every time, especially if you usually have a handful of dried fruit mid-afternoon or go wild throwing it onto your porridge in the morning.

63. WIN WITH BUTTERFLY & BACKSTROKE

Don't like running? Me neither.

That's why I don't do it. But so many people force themselves to do some type of exercise that they really don't like.

If you're a fan of swimming, then here's why you might want to get back into that swimming gear and jump in the pool.

Studies have shown that notching up the lengths several times per week can help improve your body composition, increase strength and improve your blood lipid profile.[124]

Swimming has also been found to be more effective in reducing body weight and fat distribution compared with walking.[125]

It's also a fantastic, low-impact option for people who maybe don't have the best joint health or are recovering from an injury. Swimming can also help you unwind and many find it very relaxing, especially if you get to jump into the Jacuzzi or steam room afterwards.

If you mix things up a little and vary what stroke you do, swimming is excellent for flexibility as you take many joints (like the shoulders) through a full range of motion.

If you're not a fan of swimming because you get bored easily, try swimming for a certain period of time rather than a set number of lengths. This way you're able to let your mind wander and relax, rather than focus on keeping count and remembering how many lengths you've done.

Like most training programmes or exercise regimes, it's important not to just do the same thing over and over again. Firstly, you'll get bored and, secondly, you won't progress as quickly compared with having some variety.

Try to alter your pace, use a float to work just on your legs, or get a pool buoy to do some lengths just using your arms.

》 Here's a good swimming workout for a beginner:

- 4 x 25m easy warm-up (ideally this will be freestyle/front crawl, but you can do breast stroke if you prefer)
- 2 x 25m with a float, so you just use your legs.
  Rest 20 seconds between lengths.
- 2 x 25m with a pool buoy, so you just use your arms.
  Rest 20 seconds between lengths.
- 4 x 100m with 30 seconds rest between each 100m.
- 2 x 25 fast swim. Rest 30 seconds between each length.
- 4 x 25m cooldown.

Total = 750m, 30 lengths of a 25m pool

TAKE-HOME HABIT

Swimming has a tonne of benefits and, if you enjoy it, it can be a great way to improve your fitness and decrease your body fat.

64. LEARN THE WEIGHT OF A PORTION OF NUTS

Nuts are a pretty sensible snack, right?

They're packed with a variety of vitamins, minerals, phytosterols and antioxidants, and studies have shown that these may help you to fight disease and live longer.[126]

Because of the protein, fat and fibre content, they're also quite satiating, meaning that they help you to feel full and fight the hunger demons.[127]

They're also often touted as a great weight-loss snack, but are they really?

I'd argue not.

Sure, they're packed with nutrients but they're also packed with calories and they're very palatable, meaning that it's quite easy to eat a lot of them in one sitting.

For example, a 25g serving of nuts (almonds, macadamias, Brazils, walnuts, or any other typical nut) comes in at around 125 to 150 calories.

That might not seem too much, but have you ever actually weighed out 25 grams? It's not a lot!

Even the individual serving packs you pick up in the supermarkets weigh 50–70g. This means you're easily getting through 250 to 400 calories all in one small snack. Add to that the fact most people won't weigh out a serving, and will simply pluck handful after handful from a big bag. It's not uncommon to get a good 1,000 calories purely from your pistachios or peanuts in an afternoon!

Another thing to be wise to is how much nut butter you slather on your toast and rice cakes. Again, because peanut/almond/cashew butters are very energy dense, it can be very easy to eat way more calories than you think you're actually eating.

Now, you'll know that the message throughout this entire book is not to exclude any food unnecessarily, and nuts and nut butters are no different. Just don't go wolfing entire packs of them because someone told you they were a healthy snack.

TAKE-HOME HABIT

If you do include them in your daily diet, please be smart: weigh out a portion, if necessary, and just apply the usual guiding principles of moderation.

65. JUMP INTO JOURNALLING

One of my favourite authors is a guy called Robin Sharma. He's written many books about success, mindfulness, productivity and all that good stuff. One of his top recommendations for becoming BIW (Best In World) or achieving NLG (Next Level Greatness) – two of his favourite acronyms – is to keep a journal.

A journal isn't like a diary. A diary is somewhere you record events or food you've eaten (as we discuss in Dial in Your Diet with a Diary on page 166); a journal is where you reflect and analyse your experiences and write down what goes on in your mind, allowing you to note down key lessons you've learned and deconstruct any mistakes you've made to try to stop them happening again.

If you had some really bad cravings, write them down and describe what you did to get over them – or if you didn't. If you had a fantastic workout, write down why it was so good. If you felt a bit down and sluggish, write down what you think caused this and how you were able to make it better.

By journalling your weight-loss journey, you'll be creating your own motivational bible which will help you tremendously.

You don't have to write an essay every day. Just set aside 5 minutes to write down what went well that day and what could be improved upon. In fact, you don't even need to do it every day: start with a weekly journal and, as you get more into it, up the frequency until you're able to do it as part of your daily routine.

» Here are some questions you could reflect upon:

- What were the best three things that happened today?
- How could I have made today better?
- What are the main roadblocks that may affect my weight loss in the next week?
- What did I do today that made someone else's day better?

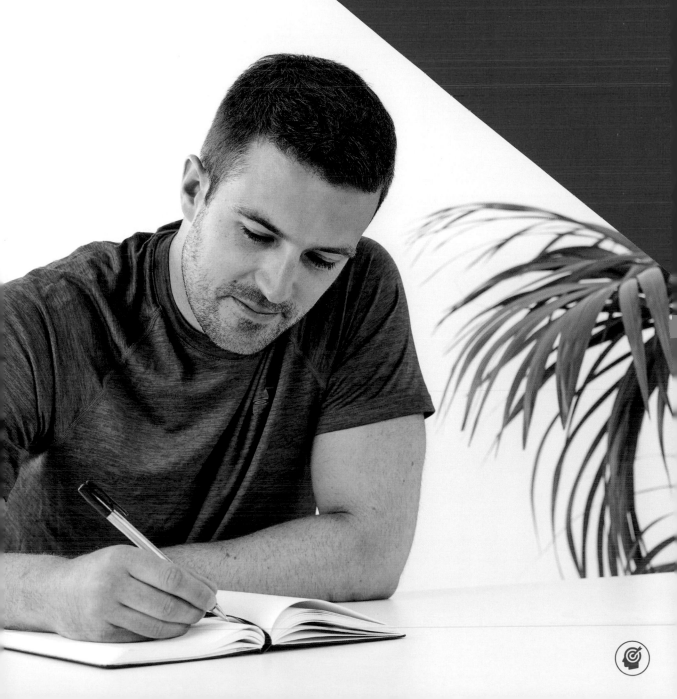

TAKE-HOME HABIT

Journalling is just part of the process of becoming more mindful of what you're eating, which has been a recurring theme throughout this book. As a minimum, try to jot down what went well and what could be improved upon each day in a notebook or on your phone.

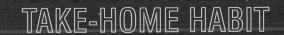

66. SCRUTINISE SNEAKY PACKAGING

Food marketers love to try and dupe you. Here are a couple of marketing tactics that you need to be aware of.

Zero-sugar sweets

Sugar-free sweets might seem like a fat loss gift sent from the gods, but here's where that old saying – '*If it sounds too good to be true...*' – really does come into its own.

All that happens here is that the sugar is replaced with sugar alcohols.

Technically, that means the manufacturers can label them as sugar-free, yet the calories and the carbs are virtually the same.

It's a sneaky trick, but one that so many people fall for.

Net carbs

If a product boldly claims to only have a certain number of net carbs, check the packaging very carefully. Net carbs are the carbs left once fibre and sugar alcohols have been subtracted. This was a bit of a fad around the Atkins and low-carb craze.

The bottom line, however, is that these non-net carbs still count, so don't be duped into thinking a food with fewer net carbs is better or lower in calories.

'Added-protein' breakfast cereals

Cereal is another food item that has fallen victim to the 'added protein, therefore it's better' fad that seems to be sweeping through the supermarket shelves.

I compared a normal breakfast cereal with the 'added-protein' version. What was the difference? A measly 3.1g! Seriously, that was it. All the other nutritional values were pretty much exactly the same.

Want an easier way to get more protein in your cereal? Add more milk. Want even more? Add a scoop of protein powder to the milk. Simple!

TAKE-HOME HABIT

Don't be fooled by fitness buzzwords plastered on packaging. Look at the ingredients on the back and see if the quantities add up and if it's worth the price.

67. ENJOY YOUR EGGS (NOT JUST FOR BREAKFAST)

Eggs are a way to win at breakfast!

They're packed with loads of nutrients and vitamins, including protein, calcium, iron, magnesium and vitamins A, B6 and B12, C and D. But no doubt you will have heard some say that eggs can be bad for your heart.

If you look at the evidence, observational studies have shown that there is no link between eating eggs and an increased risk of heart disease.[128]

In another study, subjects were asked to eat as many as three eggs on a daily basis. The result? A majority of those who participated in the study attained quite a few health benefits including weight loss and improved cholesterol levels.[129]

To yolk or not to yolk?

In the fitness world and on various 'clean-eating blogs' you'll see folk love to guzzle the egg whites while the yolks get ditched. It's a shame, because the yolks are the most nutritious part of the eggs.

Egg whites only contain water and protein, whereas the egg yolks contain almost all the nutrients and vitamins in eggs.

The yolk is also full of omega-3 fatty acids (see Go Big on Awesome Omega-3s on page 202), which are beneficial to heart health. Yes, that means the yolk has more calories, but they're also a good source of choline, lutein and zeaxanthin. Choline is crucial for the health of the heart and brain, while lutein and zeaxanthin are beneficial for the eyes.

As with everything we eat, it all comes down to moderation.

Eating a box of eggs every day is probably not a smart move.

However, having eggs a couple of times per week as a protein-packed meal is going to provide you with a nutrient hit and a nice serving of protein to keep hunger pangs at bay and help with muscle recovery, at breakfast or at any time of the day.

TAKE-HOME HABIT

Eggs are probably not the heart attack-inducing villain that some outdated publications would have you believe, but the rules of moderation still apply.

68. EAT, EXERCISE, REPEAT

You've probably heard that fasted cardio, or exercising on an empty stomach in the morning, is much better for fat loss than exercising after eating.

Roll out of bed, haul on your sports gear, grab your trainers, then hit the pavement before breakfast. Some claim this is far better for dropping those pounds than exercising later in the day.

But does it really make a difference in the grand scheme of things?

In short, no.

When it comes to fat loss, physiologically, it always boils down to calories in versus calories out. It's not dependent on what time of day you exercise, or if you do your cardio fasted or not. Because...

300 calories are 300 calories.

Let's imagine that one day you decided to head out for a run at 6AM on an empty stomach and burn 300 calories. The next day you do the same run, burn 300 calories, but this time it was after work. On both days, when you go to bed, you've still burned 300 calories, regardless of what time you exercised. Make sense?

The science supports this, too. One study in *The Journal of the International Society of Sports Nutrition* recruited 20 healthy females and split them into two groups. One group did fasted cardio for 3 hours per week, the other exercised after eating.

The result? Both groups lost weight, but there were no significant differences between the two groups.[130]

Your body doesn't know, or really care, what time of day you decide to train. The main thing is to pick a time and type of exercise that you enjoy. You should also follow a routine that you can consistently stick to.

Should you eat before exercising in the morning?

It's really down to you, but if you have the time to let the food digest, it's probably a good idea.

If possible, I usually recommend that folk eat a snack or meal 2–3 hours before exercising. It should contain a small amount of protein and some quality carbohydrates, as these will be one of your main fuel sources.

The carbohydrates you eat before exercising can top up your fuel reserves and could actually increase training intensity, thereby burning more calories compared with not eating at all.

TAKE-HOME HABIT

The idea of fasted exercise being superior for fat loss is a bit of an old-school bodybuilding myth and you're likely to have more energy in your workout if you eat about 2 hours beforehand.

69. BEWARE OF MULTI-LEVEL MARKETING

I'm not sure about you, but I've lost count of the number of times I've had someone called Karen slide into my Instagram or Facebook page with 'Hey, Scott, I've got an amazing opportunity for you. It helped me lose 30lb in just over a week... want to chat more about it?'

No, Karen. I don't want to chat more about it and neither should you!

Karen is a distributor for a multi-level marketing (MLM) nutrition company. She makes a commission if you buy some of her weight-loss products, and she'll make even more if you go on to recommend them to your friends, too. There's a load of these schemes out there and most are based on the same principles.

» Here's why you want to steer clear:

• Firstly, the people pushing these nutrition products usually have zero qualifications in nutrition. That should get the alarm bells ringing from the get-go. At an absolute push, they've attended a weekend course about the products they're selling, which focuses primarily on how to sell them, not on what goes into them or if they even work. There's a high chance they'll use sensational buzzwords like 'thermogenic', 'detoxification' and 'fat oxidising'... Terms which they don't actually understand, but who cares as long as it helps to convince you, the customer, that you've got some ailment that their product can cure?

• Secondly, your pal isn't really that fussed if you actually manage to lose weight, they just want you to buy their severely inflated shakes and potions so they can take a hefty commission. They're pretty biased.

- Lastly, many of these products aren't even that good quality. Even though you're paying two or three times the equivalent of a similar product that you could get down at your local supermarket or supplement shop, the ingredients often aren't great. For example, one of the leading MLM protein shakes uses soy as its protein choice. The problem with soy is that studies have shown that it isn't as effective at stimulating muscle recovery and repair[131] (muscle protein synthesis) as whey protein, which is the type of protein found in most protein supplements.

Another issue I have with these products is that they often contain 'proprietary blends'.

This isn't a good thing! It is a sneaky trick the supplement companies like to use. They have to tell you what ingredients they put in the blend, but they don't need to tell you how much. That means they can say their blend includes various ingredients that may have some research-based evidence behind them, like creatine, beta-alanine, caffeine, etc, but there might only be trace amounts of them in the product.

Not cool.

TAKE-HOME HABIT

Don't be tempted to shell out on a tonne of supplements sold by your neighbour or anyone else. Although their marketing pitch might be attractive, it's going to result in more heartache for you and is unlikely to result in lasting weight loss.

70. KEEP TABS ON YOUR BAR TAB

You want to find the balance between a healthy social life yet you want to lose weight at the same time.

As you know, booze isn't great if you're trying to get lean.

What's your favourite tipple?
- 220 calories in a pint of cider
- 200 calories in a pint of Guinness®
- 185 calories in a large glass of white wine
- 170 calories in a pint of beer

A few drinks can also start a spiral of events that lead to more and more calories. The pizza on the way home from the night out and then the hangover munchies the next day. Your weekly calorie deficit could be completely eradicated by a weekend session.

Ok, Scott, I get it. Limit booze, but is there a 'fitness-friendly' drink?

I wouldn't say there is a 'fitness-friendly' drink, but lower calorie drinks like gin/vodka with diet mixers are probably the least detrimental choices.

Also, if you are going to be drinking after playing some sport, drinking alcohol straight after is a pretty terrible idea.

» Here's why
It can slow down your rate of recovery, it can lead to further dehydration, it limits your body's ability to restore your muscles with glycogen (the fuel you've used up in training) and it slows down the muscle recovery process known as protein synthesis.

If you're going to the pub after playing some sport, make sure you drink plenty of water and try to have a protein and carbohydrate recovery meal before drinking.

But here's the deal – I'm not going to be a total bore; you know that moderation is always key.

The occasional pint or glass of wine is probably not going to make a huge difference to your physique and you can even track it on a calories tracker tool if you're following the tip in Dial in Your Diet with a Diary (page 166).

But if you're trying to get leaner, healthier and fitter, then regular drinking isn't going to get you closer to where you're trying to be. My recommendation would be to cut out mid-week drinking altogether.

TAKE-HOME HABIT

If you drink at the weekend, set a limit and stick to it. If you're out with mates, drink light-coloured spirits – they're lower in calories. If you're worried about peer pressure, order water when you get the round in; nobody will notice!

71. TAKE TWO-FROM-FOUR WHEN EATING OUT

Going out for dinner when you're trying to lose weight doesn't have to be the knee-shaking, fear-inducing event that many make it out to be.

Unfortunately, it's all too common to see 'fitstagrammers' posting about how they can't go out for dinner because they don't know what's in the food and they can't track the macros (see Fill up on Fibre-Rich Food on page 70). Get a grip! This isn't normal. Getting to banter with friends while eating tasty food that you don't have to cook that isn't served from a plastic box should be a treat that many should relish.

The good news is that you can easily eat out and still make healthy choices.

One guideline I like to follow is the **Two-From-Four Rule**.

Your four choices are a starter, main course, pudding and an alcoholic drink. You can pick any two. It's a simple way to keep your calories in check and not go overboard.

Another tip is to pick a source of lean protein, and eat this first.

Your lean protein could be chicken breast, a juicy rump or sirloin steak, a nice piece of fish, or, if you're a veggie, some eggs, soy, or even beans.

The reason why this works is pretty cool. Protein is the most filling macronutrient, so by eating your protein before your carbs (like rice, chips or pasta,) you'll feel full and want to eat less of the more calorie-dense stuff.

If you do want to indulge a little after your protein, by all means go for it. But it's guaranteed you won't want to eat as much and will consume fewer calories than if you went all in on the carbs first off.

Another suggestion could be to ask for veggies instead of starches, or at least ask for a side salad or extra veggies. Lastly, eat slowly, and make conversation as much as possible, so you delay the digestion process and feel fuller.

TAKE-HOME HABIT

If you're worried that eating out is going to sabotage your progress, don't be. Whether you eat out for enjoyment, or because you have to for work, it's not an issue; just make smart choices.

72. FIRE UP FAT BURNING WITH A FAST FINISHER

You're sweaty, hot, sore, potentially hangry (hungry + angry) and counting down the reps until your workout is done. This is the perfect time to add a 'finisher'. 'I love finishers'... said no one, ever.

As horrid as they may be, finishers are a great fat-loss tool that you can bolt on to the end of your workout.

In short, a finisher is usually a set or two of something quite intense at the end of the workout to burn up any gas you've got left in the tank. Before you start, don't try to be a hero. Don't add in a finisher after every workout, otherwise you'll burn out and probably burn your gym card so you don't have to put yourself through it again!

Here are 6 of my favourite finishers for you to try:

» Battle Rope Blast
Grab hold of the battle ropes and pummel your arms non stop for 30 seconds. Take 30 seconds' rest then do it again. Try to perform 3–6 working sets.

» Box Jumps Blitz
Face a soft box (your choice of height), squat down then jump explosively onto the top of the box then step off slowly then repeat. You can increase the height of the box as you get better. Aim for 10–20 reps.

» Kettlebell Fat Killer
Grab a kettlebell and do 5 upright rows, 10 goblet squats, 15 two-handed swings. See how many you can complete in 5 minutes.

(cont.)

TAKE-HOME HABIT

Finishers can be a great way to give your metabolism a further boost at the end of a workout. Think about adding in a couple per week but don't do them every session.

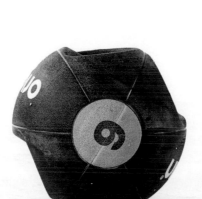

FIRE UP FAT BURNING WITH A FAST FINISHER

» **Medicine Ball Madness**

Squat down, pick up a medicine ball, stand up while raising the ball above your head then slam it down onto the ground. Jump over the ball forwards, then backwards, pick it up then slam it again. See how many of these you can do in a minute. If you're feeling brave, take a rest for 30 seconds and go for another minute.

» **The Ladder of Doom**

Pick a dumbbell isolation exercise (like a dumbbell curl, lateral raise, hammer curl, triceps kickback, etc). Start with a weight that allows you to do around 10–12 reps. Once you've done the first set, move down a weight and do the same again, then the same again until you're right down to the little dumbbells.

» **5-10-15**

Do 5 pull-ups, 10 press-ups, 15 squats (no weight). Then rest. See how many rounds you can complete in 5 minutes.

73. CURB YOUR CARBS AFTER 6PM

Hold your horses! I thought 'no-carbs after 6PM' was a myth!

Let me explain. The idea that carbs eaten after 6PM become more fattening than carbs eaten before 6PM is not true.[132]

300 calories from carbs will always be 300 calories, regardless of when you eat them. And, as you know, body composition changes are determined by calories in vs calories out. That's what we've been talking about in this book. However, what we've also been talking about is how you can develop habits to reduce your overall calorie intake... Dropping carbs after 6PM could help you do this.

» Here's why

Let's say that 50% of your dinner plate usually has some kind of carbohydrate. A large plate of pasta, a hunk of garlic bread, a load of potatoes. This could easily be 300+ calories.

What would happen if you dropped those carbs and swapped them for either more protein or, even better, more veg? Exactly – you'd make a big calorie reduction yet you'd still get plenty of food, especially if you piled on the veg.

What about after dinner? If you have a biscuit with your coffee and you can't have carbs, what do you do? You'd perhaps have some natural yoghurt for pudding instead. Then there's that pre-bed snack of some toast. No carbs means you've got to find a suitable swap for those, too.

See where I am going with this?

TAKE-HOME HABIT

I want to reiterate that carbohydrates eaten after 6PM do not become more fattening, but dropping carbs after 6PM could be an easy way to slash your calorie intake for the day.

74. DESIGN DINNER WITH THE RULE OF QUARTERS

This is a ridiculously simple brain tattoo that you can use any time you're making a meal. It works well if you're cooking at home, if you're out for dinner or if you're at a buffet.

One quarter of your plate should be a lean source of protein (chicken, turkey, fish, venison, etc).
One quarter of your plate should be a carbohydrate source.
Two quarters (half) of your plate should be green veg.

Simple.

Why does this work?

It's a simple way to reduce your calories without compromising on food volume. When you think about an average person's dinner plate, about 80% of it will be the carbs: lots of pasta, a mound of rice or a huge hunk of bread. Now there is nothing wrong with any of those foods, it's just the portion size that's the problem. The rest of their plate will have some protein, little (if any) veg, and probably some kind of rich sauce, too. Added all together, it's a sh*t load of calories.

Compare that average plate with one made using the Rule of Quarters. When you fill the plate with green veg, you're adding a high-volume, low-calorie, very nutrient-dense food group to the plate and that doesn't leave that much room for anything else.

Green veg becomes the lead actor with the carbohydrate becoming the understudy, thereby reducing the number of calories on your plate. It will also help you level up your plating skills worthy of a #FoodPorn Instagram shot, as fresh and colourful vegetables will make any dinner look more appealing.

Use some garnishes, too, even if you're not trying to be the next food blogger, a handful of chopped parsley on top of most dishes will help to instantly level-up your presentation and may even help win over some fussy eaters in the household.

Another tip that works if you're at a buffet is to fill up your plate with the lowest-calorie items first.

Start with the veg, then go to the protein then the carbs, followed by any sauces. By the time you get to the chips and roast potatoes, you'll be struggling to find room.

TAKE-HOME HABIT

The Rule of Quarters is a simple model to follow that will help you create a healthy dinner plate every time.

75. WIN AT WEIGHT LOSS WITH WATER

Roll out of bed, neck a glass of water and you'll eat fewer calories at breakfast.

One study to show this found that the group who drank a 500ml glass of water beforehand ate around 13% fewer calories at breakfast versus those who didn't have the water.[133]

Another study found that having water with a meal helps to increase feelings of satiety and decrease hunger, too.[134]

Water helps you win: another study[135] found that habitual water drinkers consumed around 9% fewer calories over the course of a day compared with those who didn't drink much water; and another found that water helped people lose weight independent of any changes in diet or activity.[136]

Okay, last bit of water science for you. Researchers in Germany had a 'water intervention' in two schools where they installed drinking fountains and the kids had a couple of lessons about the benefits of staying hydrated. The results? A 31% lower risk of being overweight.[137]

That's pretty impressive!

Let's put it into action. How can you drink more water?

Here are a couple of simple tips

>> Set a water target for each day and track it
MyFitnessPal® lets you do this.

>> Buy a sexy looking water bottle that you keep on your desk and fill it up regularly
If the water is right there, you'll drink it. If you have to go to the water fountain every time to fill a little plastic cup, you won't.

(cont.)

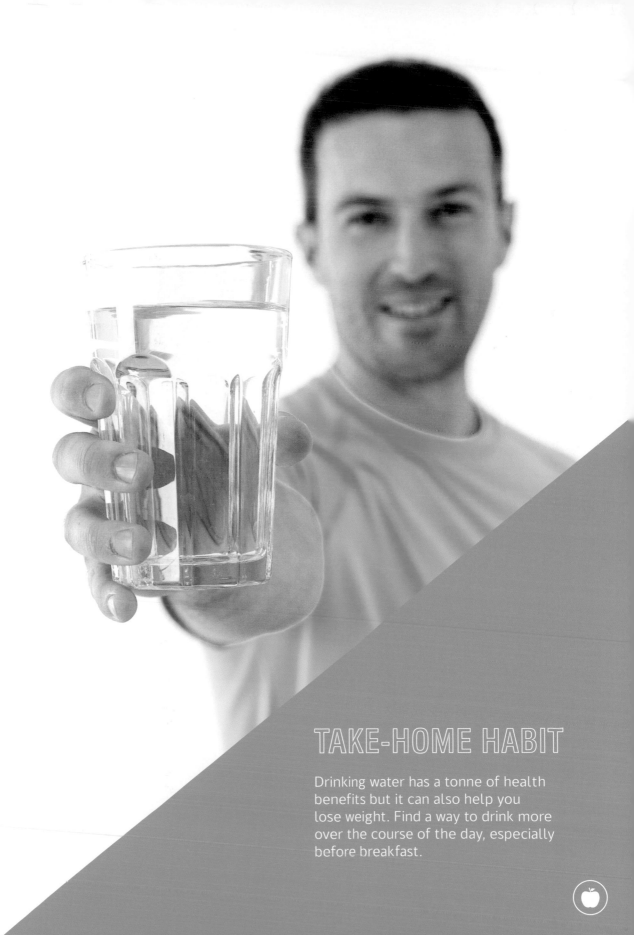

TAKE-HOME HABIT

Drinking water has a tonne of health benefits but it can also help you lose weight. Find a way to drink more over the course of the day, especially before breakfast.

WIN AT WEIGHT LOSS WITH WATER

>> Make it a routine
Every time you leave your desk, stop by the drinking fountain.

>> This is one of my favourites: get a 2l bottle of water
Get a marker pen, draw a line round the circumference of the bottle a quarter of the way down and write 'mid-morning'; do the same halfway down and write 'lunch'; finally, three-quarters of the way down write 'mid-afternoon'. This is a simple way to keep on top of your intake and, before you know it, you'll be 2 litres to the good.

76. STAY CLEAR OF ADVICE ON SOCIAL MEDIA

'Your stomach shouldn't be a waste basket.'
'Don't reward yourself with food; you're not a dog.'
'This month's diet is next month's body.'

... and other memes, 'fitspiration' and garbage titbits of 'clean eating' nutrition advice are rife on Instagram.

The big problem with Instagram and other social media sites is that they provide platforms and a voice to people who have zero nutrition or fitness qualifications. A large following can be perceived as badge of authority. The information they spout can often be incorrect (based on their opinion rather than evidence), impractical and sometimes dangerous.

This isn't to say that all Instagrammers post bad advice – there are many who post evidence-based and helpful content.

However, photo and video-sharing services enable people to display a highlight reel of their life. You see what they want you to see. You see their green smoothies. You see their toned tummies. You see them eating their chia seeds and goji berries. You don't see that it took them 100 attempts to capture the light perfectly on their abs. You don't see that they make an income from doing endorsements. You don't realise that their 21-day fat-burning plan ebook was written by someone on Fiverr.

Social media is all smoke and mirrors.

TAKE-HOME HABIT

Be careful of who you follow on social media. If you want some suggestions of people who post good content, find me (@ScottBaptie) and follow who I follow.

77. TAKE ON A TOUGH CHALLENGE

In recent years there's been a boom in weekend warriors getting down and dirty in the mud all over the country as they put themselves through military-style assault courses.

Since 2010, over 2.5 million people have taken part in the original Tough Mudder in over 6 countries and raised millions for charity in the process.[138] These adventure races are generally around the 10-mile mark and feature an array of obstacles that you have to haul yourself up, over and through while scrambling through mud pits, dodging icy pools of water and flaming hay bales.

If this sounds like your idea of hell on earth, well, that would be mission accomplished if you asked the creators. Anyway, these events can be a winner if you're trying to lose weight.

» Here's why

Firstly, it's a clear, date-defined goal that gives you purpose to get your bum into the gym and to strap on the trainers and pound the pavement. Sometimes, when we're just exercising for the sake of exercising, it's easy to pick your favourite exercises, to go easy or not to even bother to show up. When you commit to 'training', rather than 'exercising', workouts take on a new purpose.

In order to complete these events, you need to actually train for them. Even if you just walked at one of these events, you probably wouldn't mange to finish unless you put some work in beforehand.

Aside from the cardiovascular fitness involved, you need to have a reasonable level of strength, too. My tip is to make sure you're doing plenty of 'pulling exercises' in the gym as these will help you haul your ass over the walls and up the ropes that you'll face on the course. Rowing variations like a barbell or dumbbell row are helpful, as are pull-downs or pull-ups, if you can manage them.

Secondly, there is a great sense of camaraderie at these events. You generally need to work in a team; you can't be a lone wolf. This means that it's a great idea to train with a buddy in the run-up to it, too. You'll be able to hold each other accountable, motivate each other, and I always find that having someone to chat to when training makes it considerably more enjoyable than going solo, especially if that training is outside in the cold and the rain.

When you complete the event there is a huge sense of achievement. It's not about the time or the medal, it's about knowing that you worked your ass off for several months, probably lost weight in the process, and completed something that you never thought you could!

TAKE-HOME HABIT

Obstacle races provide a great incentive to get into the gym and help with adhering to a training plan. They can help you get stronger, fitter and leaner.

78. DIAL IN YOUR DIET WITH A DIARY

This is one of the easiest tools you can pull out in your fat-loss tool box. It's one of those ones that will make you say, 'Scott, that's too easy, it won't work for me'.

You don't need to consciously make any changes to what you eat. You don't need to change what you drink and it doesn't involve any exercise. Sounds too good to be true, right?

All you've got to do is to keep a food diary. Yup, that's all. You just need to write down EVERYTHING that you eat or drink and studies show that it can help you lose weight.

One study found that 69% of participants lost weight when they kept a food diary for 3 or more days per week[139] and the average weight loss was 13lb!

How does it work?

Food diaries help you lose weight simply because you become more mindful of what you're eating, which is key! Researchers found that among British people who tried to lose weight in the last year, 35% had no idea how many calories they ate on an average day![140]

Food diaries also let you see how much or how little of certain foods you eat and they're fantastic for helping you identify triggers that may cause you to overeat.

'I didn't realise I ate so few vegetables.'

'I thought I ate more protein than that.'

'When I don't eat for hours I always eat too much in the next meal.'

Here's how to make a food diary work for you:

» Be honest
Don't try to cheat yourself by writing down one or two crisps if you ate the whole bag. If you're not going to be honest, there isn't any point doing this. Include your weekends or your 'bad days', too – don't just write down days when you've 'been really good' as that will create a false picture of what's actually going on.

» Write as you go
Studies show that we're really bad at guessing what we ate and we usually underestimate the calories in meals.[141] Don't wait until the end of the day to write your diary – make a note on your phone or write it down as soon as you eat something.

» Be accurate
Try to be as accurate as you can when writing down portion sizes and try and include quantities. It doesn't have to be an exact figure, but instead of 'steak and chips with some vegetables', try and be more descriptive, e.g. 'palm-sized sirloin steak with fat removed, ¼ of the plate with oven chips and half a bag of mixed salad'.

» The more the better
Try and keep a food diary for as many days as you can. Studies have found that folk who have a better adherence and consistently log their intake usually find this tactic more effective than those who complete their food diary once in a blue moon.[142]

TAKE-HOME HABIT

Try to keep a food diary for at least a week. Write down everything you eat and drink and it will help you spot areas for improvement, like what you could eat more of, along with foods you should probably eat less of.

79. ROCK THE ONE-SALAD-A-DAY RULE

Salads are a bit of a cliché when it comes to losing weight and the thought of eating more of them is usually as appealing as a lumpy protein shake. But before you turn over the page, stay with me.

The one-salad-a-day rule doesn't really require much explanation. It's a simple way to dramatically reduce your calories for one of your meals, most likely lunch or dinner. One salad a day.

Salads are a winner for weight loss.

But for some strange reason most people have an affinity to bags of iceberg, some cucumber and a tomato. Boring! If that's your idea of a salad, it's no wonder you're not a fan.

I'm on a quest to change your opinion of salads. They're packed with nutrients, filling if you whack in a load of fibrous greens, and low in calories, assuming you don't go mental with the olive oil and cheese toppings.

Here are a couple of my favourite salad combos:

Epic Chicken Salad of Peace
> 100g [3½oz] cooked, chopped chicken breast
> 100g [3½oz] baby leaf lettuce
> 50g [3½oz] cucumber
> 50g [3½oz] spring onion [scallion]
> 30g [1oz] black olives, pitted and drained
> 30g [1oz] sundried tomato
> 1 tsp olive oil
> 2 tbsp balsamic vinegar
> 1 tsp dried mixed herbs

Greek Salad
- large handful of chopped romaine lettuce
- ¼ cucumber, cubed
- 1 small red onion, sliced
- handful of cherry tomatoes, sliced
- handful of black olives, sliced
- 30g [1oz] feta cheese, crumbled
- 1 tsp dried oregano
- 1 tsp lemon juice
- 1 tsp olive oil
- salt and pepper to taste

BLT Salad
- 100g [3½oz] cooked, chopped, crispy bacon medallions
- large handful of chopped romaine lettuce
- ½ avocado, chopped
- ¼ cucumber, cubed
- 30g [1oz] sweetcorn
- 1 tsp olive oil
- 1 tsp apple cider vinegar
- 1 tsp honey
- salt and pepper to taste

TAKE-HOME HABIT

Salads don't have to be boring. As with any meal, you just need to be creative and find a few recipes that you like.

80. MEDITATE TO LOSE WEIGHT

When you think of meditating, the stereotype of someone sitting cross-legged doing the 'OK' sign with their hands, wrists resting on each knee, chanting 'ommmm' probably comes to mind. You probably dismissed it when someone said you should meditate to help your zen flow and align your chakras. However, meditation actually goes beyond helping you relax and there are loads of studies that have found loads of health benefits from doing so.

Stress reduction, decreased anxiety, decreased depression, improved memory, pain reduction, lower heart rate, reduced blood pressure... the list goes on and on.[143] One study also found meditation helps improve a workout and makes you more motivated to exercise.[144]

Those reasons should be good enough for you to start, but here's the icing on the cake: meditation can help with weight loss, too!

A 6-month study in 46 adults found that the group who included mindful meditation as part of their weight-loss regime lost around 2.8kg more than the group who didn't do any meditation.[145] The researchers found that meditation helped the participants to make greater improvements with their eating behaviours and they were able to show more dietary restraint.

So, how do you do it?
Get settled and find a quiet place without any distractions. Then you can get started...

(cont.)

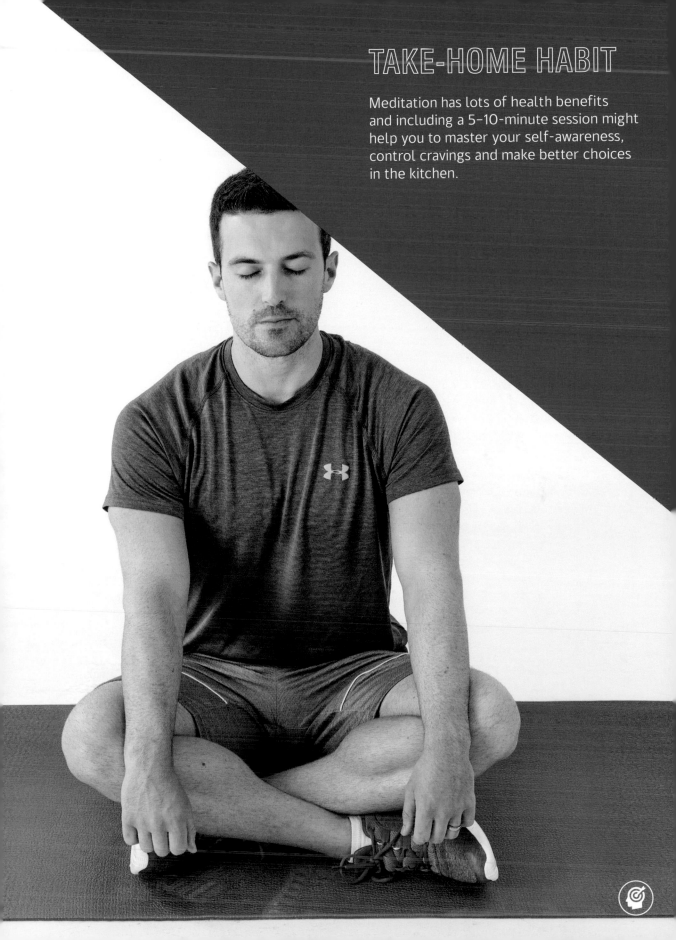

TAKE-HOME HABIT

Meditation has lots of health benefits
and including a 5–10-minute session might
help you to master your self-awareness,
control cravings and make better choices
in the kitchen.

MEDITATE TO LOSE WEIGHT

» Make yourself comfortable
Sit in a chair, keep your back upright and relax your hands
on your lap (double 'OK' signs out to the side isn't necessary).

» Breathe slowly and deeply
Don't take excessive deep breaths; just let it be a natural
process of breathing in through the nose, and out through
the mouth.

» Be aware
Are you tight or tense in any part of your body? What can you
smell? Are there any noises in the distance? Can you try to ease
the tension in tight muscles?

» Focus on your breath
Now you're becoming more relaxed, think about your breathing
and how your body moves each time you breathe in and out.
Focus on the quality of your breath and allow your mind to
wander and become still.

Try to do this for a couple of minutes each day and then go for
10 to 20 minutes. Remember to set a timer so you don't have to
keep looking at a watch. Like anything, the more you practise,
the better you'll become, and you'll find it easier to slip into a
relaxed state.

81. GET IT ON LIKE MARVIN GAYE

Ever wondered how many calories you burn between the sheets?

Researchers in Quebec, Canada, actually measured the calories burned during sex and the results looked good from a weight-loss perspective[146]. They found that on average men burn 4.2 calories per minute and women burn 3.1 calories per minute during a fumble in the jungle.

That would be 126/93 calories in 30 minutes respectively, which may be a feat in itself for some.

Almost all of the study participants reported that getting it on was way more pleasant than jumping on a treadmill.

No surprise there!

Aside from helping you to notch up a few burnt calories, there are many other benefits associated with regular sex, such as helping migraine or cluster headache sufferers. A study found that 70% of sufferers reported that sex provided moderate to complete relief of a migraine attack.[147]

Older people who have regular sex have been reported to have higher self-confidence and they report feeling between 7 to 12 years younger than they actually are.[148]

TAKE-HOME HABIT

While it may not be as effective as a workout or a run, sex is an enjoyable way to increase your calorie expenditure and will help contribute to your overall health.

82. GO EASY ON THE FATS

While the word 'fat' might strike fear into the hearts of dieters across the land, you need a certain amount of fat in your diet to stay healthy.

Although it is the most energy-dense of the macronutrients at 9 calories per gram, it has a host of important functions in the body. Fats are essential for cell growth, repair, brain function and many other key bodily functions!

As you probably already know, there are different kinds of fats. There are two high-level categories: saturated (generally from animal products like meat and dairy) and unsaturated. Unsaturated fats can be subdivided into polyunsaturated (Omega-3 and Omega-6 being the most notable ones) and monounsaturated (like the fats in nuts, seeds, olive oil, etc).

Thankfully, we seem to be moving away from the extreme zero-fat craze of the '80s and '90s, but, as with most trends, there are some in the fitness sphere who have flipped the low-fat craze on its head and are going for fats with everything and love to shout from the rooftops that 'fat doesn't make you fat'.

They would have you believe that you can eat as much fat as you like, so long as you don't eat many carbohydrates. This has led to people throwing butter and coconut oil into their coffees and smothering lard and ghee on every morsel that touches their plates.

Hopefully, by this stage in the book, you'll have realised that if something sounds a little extreme, then it's probably not going to be your best bet for long-term, enjoyable or sustainable weight loss.

In truth, the sweet spot of how much fat you should eat, as usual is going to be somewhere in the middle. As always, when it comes to weight loss, it's a case of calories in versus calories out, not specifically restricting fat or carbohydrates. There are plenty of studies that have shown that when calories are the same, it doesn't really make much of a difference to rates of weight loss whether someone is on a low-fat or low-carb diet.[149 150]

When you're in the supermarket, keep an eye on the labels.[151]

High fat means there is more than 17.5g of fat per 100g.

Low fat is when there is 3g of fat or less per 100g, or 1.5g of fat per 100ml for liquids (1.8g of fat per 100ml for semi-skimmed milk).

Fat-free is 0.5g of fat or less per 100g or 100ml.

TAKE-HOME HABIT

Try to make smart fat choices, most of the time. Eat a range of healthy fat sources and don't go crazy by adding loads of oils to foods or when cooking, as it's a sure way to end up consuming a lot of calories.

83. DOMINATE THE DIET WITH DAIRY

In recent years, dairy has developed a bit of an undeserved bad reputation.

Heard this one before?

'Cow's milk is good for baby cows, but not humans. We are the only animal that drinks the milk of another animal.'
Not true.

Several animals drink the milk of other animals, if they can get their hands/paws/beaks on it. Studies have actually found that feral cats and seagulls often steal milk from elephant seals.[152] Anyway, that's just a rebuttal that usually puts the anti-milk crew in their place.

On to the positives. Dairy has a host of benefits. For starters, it's been shown to improve body composition, reduce the risk of type 2 diabetes and minimise the risk of cardiovascular disease, particularly stroke.[153]

It's also a winner from a weight-loss perspective.

One meta-analysis (a big study of other studies) found that of the 1,278 adults studied, those who had 2–4 servings of dairy per day lost around 1.5kg more body fat than did the control group.[154]

Another found that people who ate more yoghurt experienced a greater decrease in waist circumference and body weight, too.[155]

» What does this mean for you?
Well, firstly, you should steer clear of any scaremongering blogs or documentaries that will make you think that the cows are out to get you.

It might also be a smart move to include at least one, if not two, servings of dairy in your daily diet to reap the health benefits from doing so.

Yoghurts are a winner for a mid-morning or mid-afternoon snack. If you go for the natural low-fat or natural Greek yoghurt varieties, you'll avoid all the added sugars, and the fat has been reduced to keep the calories down too.

You're likely to have seen different types of 'high-protein yoghurts'. Now, you may think that these are just a marketing ploy, but they're actually quite good and they are often quite high in protein, unlike the 'high-protein cereal' and other rubbish you'll see, as we talked about in Pile on the Protein at Breakfast (page 20). These are also especially great after a workout if you're looking for a protein-packed recovery snack.

TAKE-HOME HABIT

There is a vast amount of evidence that shows dairy boasts a load of benefits and, from a weight-loss perspective, folk who have several servings per day often lose more weight than those who don't.

84. CHUG A COFFEE BEFORE A WORKOUT

If you want to level-up your workout, chug a coffee with your pre-workout snack to boost your training intensity.

As you will have learned from this book so far, most supplements are rubbish. Caffeine is one of the exceptions!

It's a powerful stimulant – and that's why it's one of the main ingredients in popular 'pre-workout supplements' – because of its ability to delay your perceptions of fatigue and give you that buzz which can boost your workout or help get you through a gruelling run.

Caffeine has been extremely well researched and proven to improve anaerobic cardiovascular exercise, power output, aerobic exercise capacity and increase overall training volume.[156]

How much should you take?
The International Olympic Committee (IOC) suggest a small dose of around 2–3mg/kg bodyweight which is usually around 100–200mg (which you would find in a strong coffee) taken 30–60 minutes before exercise.[157]

There have also been studies that shows that caffeine can assist with weight loss as it can slightly elevate energy expenditure and it can help people to decrease their energy intake, too.[158]

More good news for caffeine.

There is a downside, however, in that the metabolism boost is only short term, and the longer-term effects aren't as impressive as people become more caffeine tolerant.

But before you go off for a flat while fix, just be careful: caffeine is highly stimulatory and is not recommended for anyone who already consumes a lot of caffeine, people with high blood pressure or heart issues. Also, it can obviously impact the quality of your sleep if taken too close to bedtime.

TAKE-HOME HABIT

If you struggle for energy before a workout, try having a strong coffee 30–60 minutes beforehand to give you a pick-me-up, which will hopefully ramp up your calorie burn, too.

85. SHRINK YOUR WAIST WITH SUPERSETS

If you're like most people, you probably have hundreds of other things you'd rather be doing than lifting weights surrounded by a mass of sweaty strangers doing the same.

Now, if you're already lifting weights, high five! It's going to help you get stronger, more powerful and leaner.[159] But here's a tip for you: add some supersets to your workout.

A superset is when you perform two exercises, back to back, without a rest. For example, you might do a set of bench presses then immediately do some pull-ups before taking a rest. Why is this effective? Well, for starters, you're going to be lifting a greater volume in less time, and this is a good thing if you want to get in and out of the gym[160] more quickly. Secondly, supersets increase the calories you burn per minute and your blood lactate, and they increase EPOC (Excess Post-Exercise Oxygen Consumption),[161] which is the calories you burn after exercise.

» There are two main types of supersets you can do:

- Antagonistic supersets work a muscle in the first exercise then its opposite in the second. For example, biceps and triceps or back and chest. This is advantageous as one study found that no rest, or a very short rest (30 seconds), between sets increased output more than a longer rest period.[162]

- Agonist supersets pair exercises that work the same muscle group. For example, dumbbell biceps curls and barbell biceps curls.

Personally, I am not a fan of agonist supersets. Yes, you may feel like you're burning more calories because your heartrate will increase because they're hard to do but you'll end up lifting less total volume per session. That isn't a good thing. If you were to take a rest between the two exercises, you would likely be able to perform more reps of the second exercise.

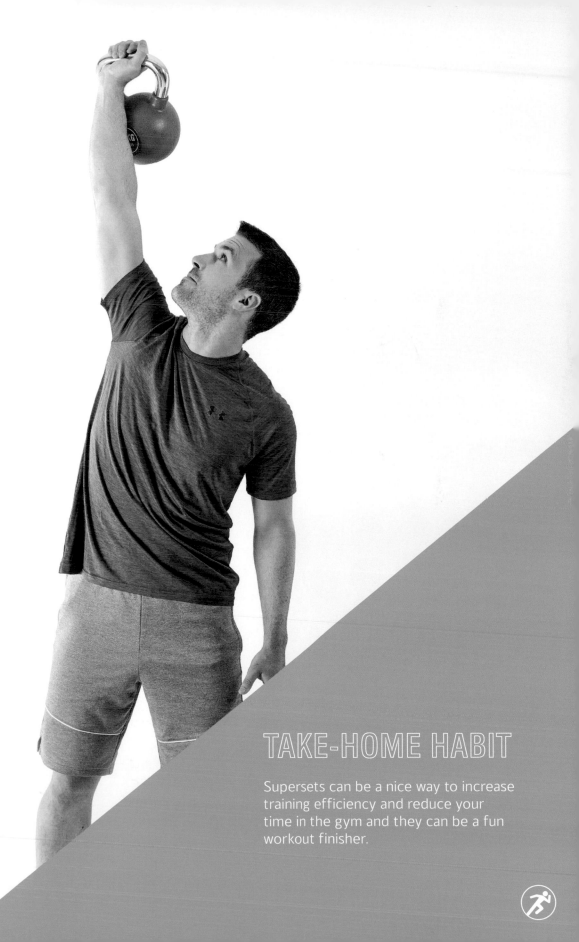

TAKE-HOME HABIT

Supersets can be a nice way to increase training efficiency and reduce your time in the gym and they can be a fun workout finisher.

86. GET SOME JELLY IN YOUR BELLY

Got a sweet tooth? Grab a no-added-sugar jelly (or a jell-o if that's your thing).

If I've got a sugar craving, then scoffing a jelly is one of my favourite sugar-craving busting hacks.

First off, they taste like birthdays.

Secondly, there are next to no calories in one of these pots. Zero sugar, 1g carbs and around 5 calories. Absolute winner here. They're great for minimising sugar cravings and they're similar to other artificially sweetened foods and drinks in that they can help improve dietary adherence.

They're a classic example of a high-volume, low-calorie food, which are great tools to have in your lunchbox when you're in a fat-loss phase.

What about the sweeteners? I covered this in Cure Cravings with Diet Drinks (page 16), but here's the summary from a review paper about aspartame (a common artificial sweetener) in the *Regulatory Toxicology and Pharmacology Journal*:[163]

'... The studies provide no evidence to support an association between aspartame and cancer in any tissue... the weight of scientific evidence confirms that, even in amounts many times what people typically consume, aspartame is safe for its intended uses as a sweetener and flavour enhancer...'

» But here's the deal.

Sugar-free jellies aren't 'healthy' and there's no nutritional benefit to be had from eating them. Aside from zero calories, there are pretty much zero vitamins and minerals, but there isn't really anything particularly 'unhealthy' about moderate consumption of them either.

If you've got a craving for jelly's favourite accompaniment – ice cream – you can make a calorie-reducing switch there too. Instead of the sugar- and fat-laden ice cream, you could have some sorbet or frozen yoghurt. The sugar content is about the same, but the latter two have a fraction of the calories, which, as you know, will help contribute towards your calorie deficit.

TAKE-HOME HABIT

Swapping from a sugar-laden snack to one of these jellies is going to reduce your overall calorie intake and will help you to eradicate a sugar craving.

87. PREPARE FOR AN ALIEN INVASION & EAT WELL

In the event of a pending natural disaster like a hurricane, tornado, flood or alien invasion, we're told by the powers that be to stock up on emergency foods to tide us over for a few days. I'd also suggest you take the same approach when you're trying to lose weight. No, really!

Let me paint a picture for you. You've had a busy day at work, traffic was terrible and the weather was dire. You still managed to get to the gym (high five!) but now you've arrived home at 8PM, tired, sore from the squats and your stomach is practically eating itself. Then you're hit by the realisation that you forgot to nip into the shops to get your groceries and you've got no meals in the freezer.

When faced with this dietary disaster, it can be all too common for people to throw in the towel and either order a greasy, calorie-loaded takeaway or just create a random concoction of bits they find in the cupboard like cheese and crackers with a side of toast, crisps and half an Easter egg.

However, if you've got an emergency food stash then you can still cook up a tasty and healthy plate of scoff to tide you over.

Some essentials that I often suggest people keep at hand: tinned tuna, tinned chicken (yes, it's a thing), frozen vegetables, tinned vegetables, tinned soup, packets of rice with the spices and veg in them already, beef jerky, nuts, frozen berries.

Frozen vegetables are not only an emergency food staple but they're also a great idea for folk who live on their own and want to keep their food waste down.

'I thought frozen vegetables weren't that good. Surely fresh is best?'

The good news is that's not true. Fresh foods often lose their nutrients quite soon after they've been harvested but fruits and vegetables that are frozen very shortly after they've been picked are able to preserve their nutrients for much longer. Researchers in California did a study to check this and they found no difference in the nutrient quality of the fresh or frozen varieties in the 8 different fruits and vegetables they tested.[164]

Another benefit of frozen veg is that it's also usually a much cheaper option, too!

Win win for the frozen veg!

TAKE-HOME HABIT

Keep a stash of emergency foods like tinned meat, soups and frozen vegetables in the event that your supermarket shop slips your mind. You can have a healthy meal without calling for a number 32 with extra spicy sauce and prawn crackers.

88. STAND MORE TO BURN MORE

This is probably one of my favourite fat-burning hacks if you work in an office. It's extremely easy to do and folks generally have no idea how effective it can be.

On average, someone who is around 80kg will burn 134 calories sitting compared with 206 calories while standing.

That's almost a 55% increase![165]

Other studies have shown that prolonged sitting may increase colon and breast cancer risk[166], and standing can improve cardio metabolic health.[167]

It's so easy to reap the benefits.

All you have to do is schedule some standing time into your day. This shouldn't be hard to do given that we office workers spend an average of 6 hours sitting behind our screens![168] If you've got a height-adjustable desk, you're off to a flyer already. If you don't, you can buy an adjustable work station that sits on your desk and you can raise or lower it so you can stand and work at the same time.

If you're going to give this one a go, don't try to stand for the entire day at work – you'll get sore and you'll pack in this habit quicker than you can say, 'This is a crock of sit'.

Start off slowly

Stand for the first 20 minutes when you get to the office, add standing blocks into your diary, stand for 10 minutes every half hour, stand after every cup of coffee you have, etc. Create a routine and work on it.

Make sure you adjust your screen and that your mouse and keyboard are positioned so they're comfortable to use.

» Another tip I love...

Try to get your office to embrace huddle meetings if your meeting is due to last for less than 15 minutes. Everyone stands. You get the benefits of standing and they're more efficient, too, as folk don't waste time with small talk and waffling as they want to get back to their chairs.

Also, if you've got a one-to-one meeting with someone and you don't need computers or papers, ask them if you could chat while you walk and head outside.

TAKE-HOME HABIT

Standing is a simple, sweat-free and easy way to increase your calorie expenditure, improve your posture and increase your life expectancy.

89. SLURP SOME SOUP TO SATISFY THE STOMACH

If you're not particularly a fan of boring green vegetables then soup can be the ace up your sleeve to fight off hunger and battle the bulge. Often forgotten about as a source of veggies, soup is a quick and easy way to cram masses of nutrients into a bowl of deliciousness.

Not only is soup extremely nutritious but it can also help you lose weight.

Researchers at Penn State University found that when diners started their meal with a bowl of soup, they consumed 20% fewer calories compared to when they just went straight for the main course.[169] Interestingly the researchers found that it didn't make much of a difference if the soup was blended or chunky; it still had the same effect on controlling calories.

Soup is a saviour if you're trying to lose weight. Because of the water content it's a classic high-volume, low-calorie food that will help you to feel full without consuming a load of calories in the process. Obviously there are exceptions; you don't want to be throwing in a load of cream or frying all the vegetables in a stick of butter but being the smart cookie that you are, you will have deduced this already.

For fussy eaters, soups can be a great way to sneak a load of vegetables that they wouldn't usually like into their system, especially if the soup is blended. It's easy to cook in bulk and it makes a fantastic, warming mid-morning or mid-afternoon snack.

Here's a favourite of mine. It serves around 4 people and the calories are just under 200 per portion.

Roast Vegetable & Sweet Potato Soup

  3 [bell] peppers, chopped
  2 garlic cloves, chopped
  2 sweet potatoes, finely chopped (so they cook quickly)
  1 tbsp olive oil
  2 red onions, quartered
  1 carrot, chopped
  1 tbsp balsamic vinegar
  2 tbsp mixed herbs
  1 litre [4 cups] vegetable stock

Preheat an oven to 200°C/400°F. Roughly chop all of the vegetables and place on a baking tray. Drizzle the olive oil and balsamic vinegar over the vegetables and roast in the oven for 20–25 minutes, or until cooked. Be sure to give them a shake/stir halfway through.

Once the veg is cooked, remove from the oven and tip into a large pan. Add the stock and simmer for 15 minutes. After 15 minutes, blend with a hand blender and serve.

TAKE-HOME HABIT

Soup can be a fantastic low-calorie, high-volume food that can help you to fight the hunger demons! Think about making a big batch of soup once a week so you've got some emergency portions in the freezer and a few meals for the week ahead.

90. EAT THE FOOD YOU LIKE!

If you've been on a 'classic' restrictive diet in the past, there is a high chance that you will have forced yourself, in a bid to be 'good', to quickly neck a few foods or glasses of goop that quite frankly made you want to vomit.

Healthy eating shouldn't be associated with boring, bland or vomit-inducing foods.

When you're implementing the tips in this book, please only eat foods that you actually like to eat. If you constantly force-feed yourself kale, sardines, avocado or any other 'healthy food' that someone said was good for you but you can't stand, you're eventually going to be defeated.

Studies have proved this.

'Regardless of assigned diet, 12-month weight change was greater in the most adherent. These results suggest that strategies to increase adherence may deserve more emphasis than the specific diet.'[170]

In other words, if you like what you're doing, you'll stick with it!

So how can we make this change to your diet different from all the others? Well, we're not talking about 'good' or 'bad' foods and you shouldn't have to eat stuff that you don't like. This book is to show you how to make small changes that, over time, will produce spectacular results; it's not about making extreme, unpleasant or unrealistic changes that you only follow for a few weeks before going right back to square one again.

This isn't to say that you shouldn't at least try and expand your palate. If you're traditionally someone with a vegetable aversion, is it because you always boil your broccoli or steam your spinach? If so, play around with different cooking methods. If you're not a fan of vegetables, try making some soups (see Slurp Some Soup to Satisfy the Stomach on page 188), try roasting vegetables (one of my favourite methods), or add in more vegetables to recipes you already like. For example, pop some extra carrots into fajitas or wilt some spinach into a Bolognese. Seriously, spinach is one of those foods that disappears into next to nothing but it's still loaded with fibre and packed with minerals and vitamins A, C and K, to name a few.

If you've never been a fish-fan, try using it in a dish that packs lots of flavour to hide the fishy taste that you might not be keen on. Fish curries or a tuna chilli are great recipes that are fantastic ways to introduce people to fish, as is a tender tuna steak that's been marinated in some delicious herbs and spices before being chargrilled on the BBQ. Yum!

TAKE-HOME HABIT

The goal is to get into the best shape you've ever been in, while having the most fun and eating the tastiest foods in the process! Don't force-feed yourself foods that you really don't like, no matter how healthy someone says they are.

91. #FOODPIC #YUM #TWEETWHATYOUEAT

Instagram is the place to go if you're a budding food stylist and photographer. Thanks to their crafty filters, you can transform a simple plate of slop into an artistic masterpiece worthy of a featuring in a lifestyle magazine. Photographing food has become the norm and people seem to love sharing what features on their dinner plate. I was out for dinner recently at one of the top-rated restaurants in Scotland and even they had a bit on their menu with top tips on how to snap your supper! How previous generations were able to eat healthily and lose fat without photographing every morsel they ate, I have no idea.

The good news is that photographing your food is actually a proven way to lose weight.

Researchers at the University of Wisconsin-Madison found that switching from a written food diary/journal (see Dial in Your Diet with a Diary on page 166) to a photographic one had a greater impact on attitudes and behaviours associated with food choices.[171]

A photographic food diary provides a lot more detail than a written one; it captures the whole meal, including any sides and sauces which can often be missed when we write it up. It's also quicker to whip out the phone and grab a pic compared with writing down every item, and the easier something is and the more convenient, it means we're more likely to stick with it.

There are several food photo journal apps that you can download to make this process even easier.

Another study[172] found that food can taste better when you take a picture of it. Researchers found that when participants were told to take a picture of their healthy meal, their taste perceptions increased and they reported finding it more enjoyable. This is also because by delaying eating, we're given more time to think about the food, the taste, the smells, so that when we actually eat it, we find it more gratifying.

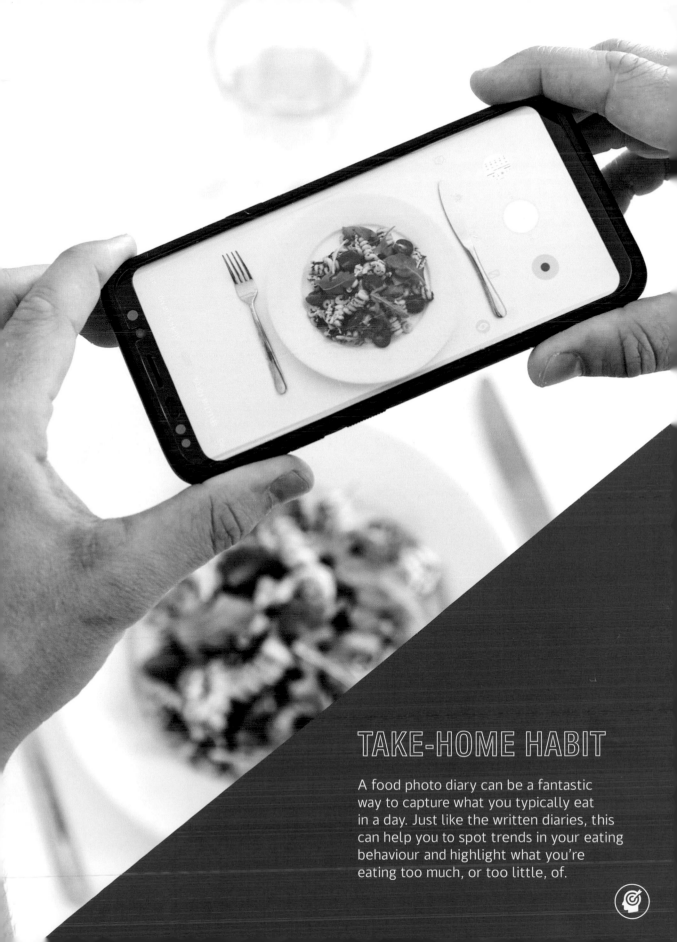

TAKE-HOME HABIT

A food photo diary can be a fantastic way to capture what you typically eat in a day. Just like the written diaries, this can help you to spot trends in your eating behaviour and highlight what you're eating too much, or too little, of.

92. PIMP UP THE PLATE WITH PROTEIN

Looking for a nifty trick to ignite your fat burning? Something that will help you to burn fat, minimise muscle loss and blunt hunger?

It sounds too good to be true and your BS detector is probably going off on overdrive, but seriously, this is legitimate. It's extremely accessible, you can get it in almost every supermarket, it's safe for kids and it's probably already found its way into your kitchen...

**What is this miracle food? I hear you cry.
Protein, of course.**

When we're trying to lose weight, it can be tempting to rush off and try all the extreme diets, detoxes, fads, pills and potions in a bid to get that dieting edge. We're often so keen to focus on the minutiae that we forget about nailing the basics first. In the hierarchy of importance, eating enough protein is going to make a significantly greater impact on your waistline compared to stressing over supplements or manipulating meal frequency.

In one year-long study of men and women, folk who had 1.6g protein per kilo of bodyweight per day lost more body fat compared with the group who ate 0.8g/kg/bw/d.[173]

One of the main benefits is that protein can help keep hunger pangs at bay. When you eat it, certain hormones are released that send messages to your brain telling it that you're nice and full. Protein also has a high 'thermic effect', meaning that your body uses more energy to digest it, compared with burning fat and carbohydrates.

Another benefit is that a higher protein intake can help you hold on to muscle. This is a good thing, even if you don't want to look like a bodybuilder! Generally, when someone talks about losing fat, the end goal is to look healthy, full of life and athletic, rather than skinny. Protein can help you to hold on to muscle, which decreases when people lose weight.

A simple way to increase your protein intake is to aim to include it with every meal – lean meat, fish, low-fat dairy, eggs, beans, pulses and some protein powders, like whey protein or soy protein, are all good sources.

When gauging how much protein you need, you don't need to get the scales out at each meal (unless you're tracking macros; see Master Macros with Flexible Dieting on page 50 for more) – just use your hands.

A fist-sized serving of chicken or beef is a good measure or a flat-hand-sized piece of fish, turkey or pork steak. The bigger you are, the higher your protein intake will be, so roughly using your hand size is going help to get you started.

TAKE-HOME HABIT

Including a wide variety of protein is beneficial for your body. It will help you to lose weight and also help to keep your diet interesting.

93. CA CANNY* WITH THE COCONUT OIL

Coconut oil is all the rage, but before you go lathering it on everything from your hair to your stir-fries, you need to realise that many of the fat burning coconutty claims have been blown out of proportion.

However, let's start with the positives. It's actually a really good addition to your kitchen cupboard.

The main benefit is that it has a high smoke point: when you heat up an oil, the properties start to change. When an oil starts to smoke, it starts to break down and the quality of the oil decreases. Some studies[174] have shown that this oxidised fat may be detrimental to our health. Refined coconut oil, like the kind you'd get in the supermarket, has a smoke point of over 200°C. As you probably guessed, this means you can cook with it at a high temperature without it smoking. This is because coconut oil is a saturated fat which means that it's really stable and resistant to heating so it doesn't oxidise easily.

If you're cooking at high temperatures like flash-frying meat or stir-frying vegetables, coconut oil is a good bet.

On to the fat-burning claims. When people talk about coconut oil being 'fat burning', they often reference the medium-chain triglycerides (MCTs) which are found in coconut oil. One study found that MCTs did have slight metabolism-boosting properties after 7 days, but this was very short lived. After 14 days there was no improvement. Other studies have found that MCTs helped to slightly reduce the body fat of test subjects who had a BMI greater than 23, but it had no impact on folk with a lower BMI.[175]

Finally, a 2017 study in the *European Journal of Nutrition* found that coconut oil had no impact on the number of calories someone ate or the amount of fat they burned.[176]

When you look at the 'fat-burning' effects of coconut oil and MCTs as a whole, it's unlikely to have any significant impact on your waistline.

What's more, at 9 calories per gram, like any other fat, coconut oil is extremely energy dense. That means that if you're smothering vegetables in it, adding it to coffee or using copious amounts in cooking, it's not only going to have zero fat-burning benefits, but the excess calories may in fact contribute to fat gain!

*NOTE: 'ca canny' is a Scottish expression for 'go easy' in case you hadn't sussed that out yet.

TAKE-HOME HABIT

Coconut oil is great for cooking at high temperatures but it doesn't have any significant fat-burning properties that exclude it from being governed by the general principles of moderation!

94. GO FOR THE LOW-HANGING FRUIT

If you've tried unsuccessfully in the past to create healthy eating habits that last, how can you change this? Ask yourself what you could do to make it so easy to eat healthily that it doesn't make sense not to.

If you're not a fan of cooking or you have a crazily busy schedule that makes it tough to exercise and cook in the same day, here are a couple of tips to simplify the process.

Buy pre-cooked meat
Most supermarkets stock a range of pre-cooked meats that require next-to-no preparation or can be eaten cold. These include flame-grilled chicken, hot smoked salmon, tinned tuna, pulled pork, or you could even grab a hot rotisserie chicken that you don't even need to heat it up – it's good to go.

Buy done-for-you veg packs
Can't be bothered chopping? Not a problem. You can get a wide range of mixed stir-fry bags that you just throw into a wok for a couple of minutes. You can buy trays of chopped and seasoned vegetables ready to be roasted, healthy tubs of fresh soups and boil-in-the-bag vegetable medleys. There are also microwaveable pouches of grains and seeds like quinoa that make life easier.

Get the jars
Chopping garlic and peeling ginger are two cooking jobs I hate, so I don't do them. I buy jars of pre-chopped garlic and fresh ginger paste. You can get chopped chillies, roast peppers, lemongrass and lots of other fiddly vegetables that you often use in cooking that are ready for you to throw straight into the pan. Most are preserved in oil or vinegar so they last for ages in the fridge too; some also come frozen so last even longer.

Slow cook your way to success
This has been covered at length in Get into Slow Cooking
(page 34), but to reiterate, a slow cooker is an absolute kitchen
essential if you want to hack your meal prep. Bung all the meat
and veg into the pot, add some stock, seasoning and spices,
put the lid on, and 8 hours later you have several servings
of tasty food to last a couple of days or that you can freeze
(once cooled).

Order your shopping online
Can't be bothered to go shopping? For very little extra cost,
most of the major supermarkets will do your shopping and drop
it off straight to your kitchen. There are also lots of companies
that offer a meal delivery service, too – they'll post you the
specific ingredients along with a recipe card to cook each day.
Other companies will send you packs of pre-cooked food for
the entire day – snacks, main meals, the full Monty.

TAKE-HOME HABIT

In today's society, the line 'I don't have
time to eat healthily' just isn't valid thanks
to a huge range of convenience foods and
services that can take the hassle out of
healthy cooking.

95. ASK IF IT SWIMS, FLIES, RUNS OR GROWS

Sometimes when people are trying to lose weight they become fixated on labels, calories, the sugar content, how many carbs are in this, is there more than 30g of protein per serving, etc, to the extent that they actually forget about food quality. Now, I am all for people being mindful about what it is they're actually eating – it's a good idea to have a rough idea of how many calories we consume, especially when studies have shown that we regularly underestimate how many calories we do actually eat – but let's not go too far down the rabbit hole.

Sometimes we spend too much time reading the labels to determine if a food is 'healthy' and not enough time asking these questions:

- Does this food swim, fly, run or grow in a field?
- Is it lean, green or marine?
- Does it start to go off within a few days?
- Did it exist when my grandparents were children?

There are obviously exceptions to the rule, but if 80% of your diet conforms to the above, then you're probably on the right track.

When you're picking foods, try to 'eat the rainbow'. As cheesy as it sounds, variety really is the spice of life. Okay, no more clichés but, seriously, aim to include as wide a range of fresh foods as you can. This helps to cover your micronutrient (like vitamin and mineral) needs, prevents deficiencies, makes eating more interesting, forces you to try new recipes and is good for preventing meal-time apathy. Nobody wants to eat broccoli and chicken all day, every day.

Should you eat organic?

If you have the desire and money to do so, then there is no harm in buying organic food. However, the research hasn't shown that there are clear health benefits in doing so.

One of the most widely cited studies on organic food (it was a systematic review, aka a big study of other studies) concluded that:

'... the published literature lacks strong evidence that organic foods are significantly more nutritious than conventional foods.'

The lead researcher in the study stated that:

'Some believe that organic food is always healthier and more nutritious. We were a little surprised that we didn't find that. There isn't much difference between organic and conventional foods, if you're an adult and making a decision based solely on your health.'[177]

TAKE-HOME HABIT

Don't become obsessed with calories and food labels. Think about the food quality: if 80% of your intake is lean, green or marine, then you'll be getting lots of micronutrients and there's a good chance your calorie intake won't be that high.

96. GO BIG ON AWESOME OMEGA-3S

You've probably been told, read or heard that you should be eating more 'healthy fats' like omega-3. You've not been fed a yarn – this is good advice. If you've been trying to buy more salmon, mackerel, sardines, nuts and seeds to boost your healthy fat intake, then you deserve a pat on the back.

I'd love to say that omega-3s will help with weight loss, but I can't. In most of the studies looking at the effects of fish oil on body fat, it hasn't had a significant impact and it certainly can't be classed as 'fat burning'.[178] However, it would be wrong to write a book about healthy eating without mentioning them.

Although fish oils aren't going to make any difference to your waistline, here are some proven reasons why you might want to eat more of them:

They reduce the risk of cardiovascular disease
Fish oils have been shown to lower blood pressure, decrease triglycerides and the build-up of fat in the arteries.[179]

Omega-3s can help prevent depression
There is evidence that shows that people who regularly consume omega-3s are less likely to be depressed and it may even help to alleviate symptoms of depression and anxiety, too.[180]

Reduced risk of rheumatoid arthritis
In a study of 32,000 elderly women, it was found that regular consumption of fish oil (more than once per week) reduced the risk of rheumatoid arthritis by 29%.[181]

There have been other studies that show omega-3s may help reduce age-related macular degeneration, reduce the risk of dementia and improve the symptoms of schizophrenia, but the jury is out on these, and there have been more recent studies in these areas that have shown fish oil to have little effect.

However, there is still good data which shows there are positive benefits to be had from munching more mackerel. The current government guidelines recommend we aim for around 2 servings of oily fish per week.[182] If you're not a fish fan, then a fish oil supplement that provides around 0.5–1g[183] of EPA & DHA (the two most useful types of omega-3s) would help to cover your bases.

TAKE-HOME HABIT

Omega-3s have a range of health benefits and to take your diet up a notch, make an effort to include more in your diet, ideally from whole foods like oily fish.

97. KICK THINGS OFF WITH A KETTLEBELL

Kettlebells are fantastic tools to include in your fat-loss arsenal which can help you lose weight, get stronger, improve flexibility and develop mobility.[184]

The exact history of the kettlebell is unknown, although we know they originated in Russia as counterweights in markets and the Russian word for kettlebell, 'girya', first appeared in the dictionary in 1704.[185]

Fast-forward to the present day and you'll find them in almost every gym. There are entire exercise classes dedicated to training with them and there are even international competitions and worldwide kettlebell federations.

Here are some of the reasons why they're so popular:

>> They're fantastic for increasing cardio fitness
In one study, participants performed a 20-minute kettlebell workout 3 times per week doing 15 seconds of snatches with 15 seconds of rest (like a HIIT workout). After 4 weeks they had increased their aerobic capacity by 6%.[186]

>> You don't need to go to the gym or pay a membership fee
You can buy a couple of kettlebells online, then you can turn your home or garage into your own workout studio. If it's a nice day, take them outside and get some vitamin D while you're working out.

>> They're extremely versatile
There is a multitude of exercises you can do with a kettlebell, from squatting and lunging to pressing and pulling.

(cont.)

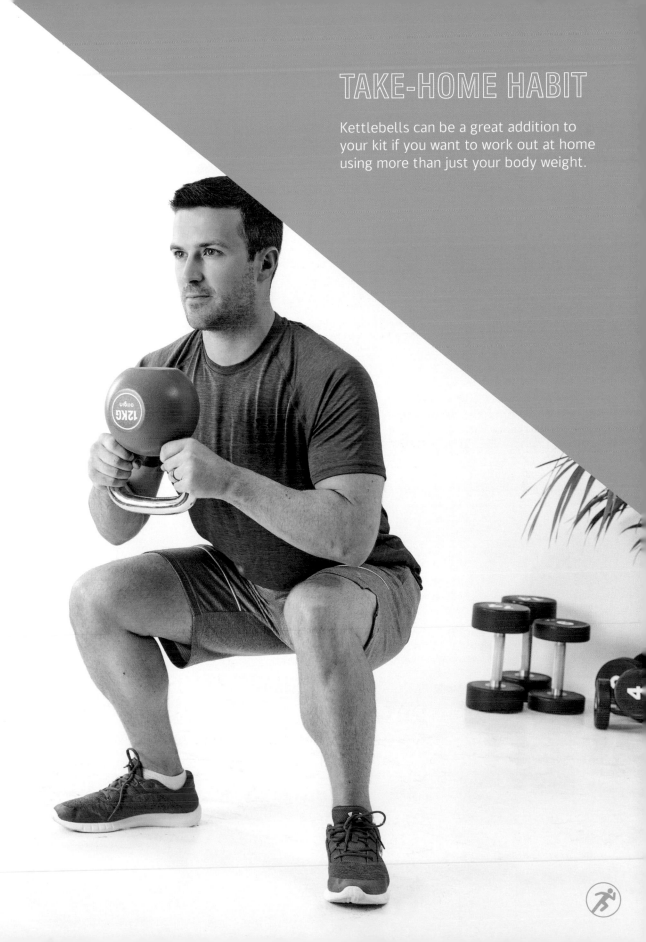

TAKE-HOME HABIT

Kettlebells can be a great addition to your kit if you want to work out at home using more than just your body weight.

KICK THINGS OFF WITH A KETTLEBELL

» It's a time saver
With a kettlebell you can train for strength, cardio and flexibility in the same workout.

» They improve coordination and movement
Many kettlebell exercises require a bit of practice before you can become really efficient with the technique. You can't just pick it up and throw it around; you have to know what exercises to do and engage your brain on every single movement.

What size of kettlebell should you get?

They range in weight from around 4kg all the way to 50kg, so it can be quite tricky to pick one to start with. For men, I'd recommend at least 10kg and no more than 25kg to start with. For women, at least 7kg and probably no higher than 20kg.

Obviously, if you want to be able to perform a wider range of exercises and ensure progression then you'll want to add to your kettlebell collection as you progress. In my garage I have kettlebells weighing 12kg, 16kg, 20kg and 30kg and I find that is perfect for what I need them for.

98. CYCLE TO WORK & CURB HUNGER

Cycling to work is a fantastic way to save cash, burn fat and do your bit for the environment.

Studies have shown that people who specifically cycle to work have increased life expectancy, a reduced risk of developing cancer and considerably increased cardio fitness![187]

It's also a fantastic solution for the 'I don't have time to exercise' people, but they're happy enough to sit in rush-hour traffic for 30 minutes to cover 5 miles... Cycling to work also ticks the box as far as the American Heart Association is concerned. They recommend that: '... *all healthy adults aged 18 to 65 yr need moderate-intensity aerobic (endurance) physical activity for a minimum of 30 min on five days each week or vigorous-intensity aerobic physical activity for a minimum of 20 min on three days each week.*'[188]

Jumping on the bike for the commute means you get two chances to boost your metabolism and not only that but exercise keeps your metabolism higher for the rest of the day, too.[189]

Cycling can also help to temporarily suppress your appetite.

When you exercise you suppress a hormone called ghrelin which makes you feel hungry and you increase PYY, another hormone, which makes you feel full.[190] This means that cycling is ideal if you find you're prone to the mid-morning munchies when you get to the office.

TAKE-HOME HABIT

If you spend hours each week sitting in the car or on the train to cover a few miles, jump on your bike instead to burn fat and save a few quid in the process.

99. GET TO GRIPS WITH 'STARVATION MODE'

If you've ever hit a weight-loss plateau and done some digging on the internet, one of the explanations you might have stumbled across is that you're not eating enough calories to lose weight and you've gone into 'starvation mode'.

This is the idea that your body will stop burning fat if you don't eat enough calories.

Let's get something straight: the reason why someone is not losing weight is NEVER because they're not eating enough calories.

As we've been chatting about throughout this book, you will ONLY lose weight if you're in a calorie deficit (eat fewer calories than you burn). If you're not losing weight, it means you're not in a calorie deficit and you're burning the same number of calories as you're eating, i.e. you're at an equilibrium.

» Here's a real-world example for you:
You know the TV programme with Bear Grylls called *The Island*? The one where people are marooned on a desert island with very little food?

Ever seen the series where they all fail to lose weight because they're 'not eating enough'? No, of course not. Many finish the show considerably lighter (and often ill-looking) due to the lack of food and increased exercise – calorie deficit at work.

On a more serious and saddening note, if the body decided to go into 'starvation mode', then the terrible plight of many who experience famine or suffer from anorexia would therefore be unexplained. The idea that someone does not eat enough to lose weight is completely flawed.

One of the best-known studies to demonstrate this was back in 1945. A researcher called Dr Ancel Keys performed the famous Minnesota Starvation Experiment.[191] Thirty-six male conscientious objectors volunteered to follow a diet of 1,570 calories for 6 months. They also walked 3 or more miles a day. Unsurprisingly, the men lost weight every week. They lost approximately 25% of their starting body weight and finished with a body-fat level of 5%.

Your body will not hold on to fat if you create a calorie deficit; it will burn it as needed for fuel until its need for energy is balanced.

(cont.)

TAKE-HOME HABIT

When you're in a weight-loss phase there are times when you might hit a plateau. There are several reasons why this could be, but it won't be 'starvation mode'. Assess what you've been doing and modify your diet or exercise as a result to get back on track.

GET TO GRIPS WITH 'STARVATION MODE'

'What about my friend who started losing weight when she started eating more food?'
Food is not the same as 'calories'.

An increase in food doesn't necessarily mean an increase in calories and vice versa. If you've been following a lot of the tips in the book so far then there's a high chance that you're eating more nutrient-dense, high-volume foods (veg, more protein, wholegrains, etc) but fewer overall calories than you did before. 'Oh, hello calorie deficit!'

» Here are some actual reasons why you might not be stuck at a plateau:

Problem: You're eating more calories than you think you are.
Solution: Keep a food diary (see page 166) or track your intake on an app to get a better idea of what you're eating.

Problem: Your NEAT has slumped (see Notch up Your NEAT the Easy Way on page 56).
Solution: Increase your step count: park further from work, get off the bus earlier, take the dog for a longer walk.

Problem: Your workout intensity has dropped.
Solution: Change-up your programme, eat a snack beforehand, work out with a buddy, change the time when you train.

100. GLUTEN-FREE ISN'T A GET-OUT

Gluten is seen as a dietary devil these days but the reality is, unless you have a medical intolerance, there's no need to avoid it.

Despite what you might have read, gluten isn't bad for you. It's just a type of protein found in wheat and some other grains and there is a high chance that you can digest it just fine.

Research shows that only 0.3–1.2% of the population suffers from coeliac disease or is allergic to wheat. Studies on gluten intolerance suggest similar figures, saying that gluten sensitivity affects less than 0.5% of the population.[192] This means that for 98% of you reading this, there is no sound reason why you would need to cut it from your diet.

Clever marketing has conditioned us to associate the label 'gluten-free' with health. The trouble with many gluten-free products is that the calorie content can actually be higher or exactly the same as their regular counterpart. With many gluten-free foods it's due to the fact the flour is usually replaced with a higher-calorie nut flour, and extra fats are added. And most of the time when you see 'gluten-free' on the label you'll also find less money in your wallet after you've been to the checkout.

Healthy eating doesn't need to be expensive or inconvenient; just read the labels and watch out for sneaky marketing tricks that are rife on food packaging.

TAKE-HOME HABIT

Gluten isn't inherently evil. The only folk who need to avoid eating it are those with a medical intolerance or allergy. Don't make healthy eating harder or more restrictive than it needs to be.

101. VISUALISE THE BODY YOU WANT

It's a technique used by sports psychologists and productivity gurus around the world and it works for professional athletes, from goalkeepers to golfers.

Visualisation is when you form an image or intention in your mind that you wish to become a reality.

Athletes use this technique to envisage the outcome of a race; they can imagine the sound of a crowd, or the thought of sinking a 50ft putt to win a golf championship, or scoring a penalty to secure the World Cup. Studies[193] have shown that this mental practice, repeated over and over, can train the body to perform the imagined skill and achieve the aim.

It's a great tactic for weight loss, too.

When I used to do fitness cover shoots and I'd be in the gym squeezing out a final rep or sweating over a cross-trainer in the quest to get leaner, I used to use visualisation all the time. When the countdown clock on the treadmill seemed to be stuck, I would conjure up the image in my mind of how I wanted to look. Why was I doing this cardio? How would my body look as a result of the hard work and focus? I'd imagine how I'd look in 12 weeks' time in peak condition. Any time I did this, the workout always seemed easier and became infinitely more enjoyable.

Studies have shown that visualisation can actually make you make better food choices, too. Canadian researchers asked 177 students at McGill University, Montreal, to eat more fruit over the next 7 days. Most of them did. However, the ones that were asked to visualise how they were going to do it (where they would buy the fruit, when they would eat it, what they would buy, how it would be prepared) ate twice as much.[194]

To utilise the power of this tactic, you can visualise the habits from this book that you're going to adopt. You're going to visualise putting them into action; you're going to visualise how you will look and feel as a result.

Spend a few minutes at the start of the day to visualise yourself resisting alcohol, going to the gym, putting on your trainers. Imagine yourself writing your food diary, think about the satisfaction you'll get from prepping your meals, think of the sounds, smells and sights you'll experience as you take a walk after work to get your 10,000 steps.

The more detailed your visions, the more likely you are to achieve them.

TAKE-HOME HABIT

Visualisation is a proven tactic from the sports psychology world that can help you to stick to your habits and win at weight loss.

YOUR NEXT STEPS

Your mission, should you choose to accept it, is to go and put some of these 101 ways into practice. You don't need to worry about 'starting on Monday'. There should be no fear about beginning 'another weight-loss program', as you've already proven that you're an action taker. You've read this book. You've shown that you're committed to positive change.

You are ready.

What's more, if all goes to plan, this will be the last time you'll ever have to start again...

Keep in touch

I'd love to hear about your success with this book. Make sure you grab your book bonus and helpful downloads here:
weightlossbook.co.uk
Then connect with me over on social media:
Instagram: @ScottBaptie
Twitter: @ScottBaptie
Facebook: /ScottBaptieFitness

FOOTNOTES

1. Brits lose count of their calories: Over a third of Brits don't know how many calories they consume on a typical day. (2016, March 9). Retrieved April 17, 2018, from http://www.mintel.com/press-centre/food-and-drink/brits-lose-count-of-their-calories-over-a-third-of-brits-dont-know-how-many-calories-they-consume-on-a-typical-day

2. United Kingdom Obesity Statistics, Figures in 2017. (2017, November 25). Retrieved April 17, 2018, from https://renewbariatrics.com/uk-obesity-statistics/

3. Polivy, J., Coleman, J. and Herman, C. P. (2005), The effect of deprivation on food cravings and eating behavior in restrained and unrestrained eaters. *Int. J. Eat. Disord.*, Dec; 38(4), 301-9.

4. Meule, A., Westenhöfer, J., & Kübler, A. (2011). Food cravings mediate the relationship between rigid, but not flexible control of eating behavior and dieting success. *Appetite*, 57(3), 582-584.

5. Baker, E., Milner, A., & Campbell, A. (2015). A pilot study to promote walking among obese and overweight individuals: walking buses for adults. *Public Health*, 129(6), 822-4.

6. Lomas, N. (2017, August 24). Global wearables market to grow 17% in 2017, 310M devices sold, $30.5BN revenue: Gartner. Retrieved April 17, 2018, from https://techcrunch.com/2017/08/24/global-wearables-market-to-grow-17-in-2017-310m-devices-sold-30-5bn-revenue-gartner

7. Willbond, S. M., Laviolette, M. A., Duval, K., Doucet, E. (2010). Normal weight men and women overestimate exercise energy expenditure. *J Sports Med Phys Fitness*. Dec;50(4):377-84.

8. Magnuson, B. A., Burdock, G. A., Doull, J., Kroes, R. M., Marsh, G. M., Pariza, M. W., & Williams, G. M. (2007). Aspartame: A Safety Evaluation Based on Current Use Levels, Regulations, and Toxicological and Epidemiological Studies. *Critical Reviews in Toxicology*, 37(8), 629-727.

9. Miller, P. E., & Perez, V. (2014). Low-calorie sweeteners and body weight and composition: A meta-analysis of randomized controlled trials and prospective cohort studies. *The American Journal of Clinical Nutrition*, 100(3), 765-77.

10. Bleich, S. N., Wolfson, J. A., Vine, S., & Wang, Y. C. (2014). Diet-beverage consumption and caloric intake among US adults, overall and by body weight. *American Journal of Public Health*, 104(3), 72-78.

11. Wansink, B., Hanks, A. S., & Kaipainen, K. (2016). Slim by Design. *Health Education & Behavior*, 43(5), 552-558.

12. Leidy, H. J., & Racki, E. M. (2010). The addition of a protein-rich breakfast and its effects on acute appetite control and food intake in 'breakfast-skipping' adolescents. *International Journal of Obesity*, 34(7), 1125-1133.

13. Weston, K. S., Wisløff, U., & Coombes, J. S. (2013). High-intensity interval training in patients with lifestyle-induced cardiometabolic disease: A systematic review and meta-analysis. *British Journal of Sports Medicine*, 48(16), 1227-34.

14. Trapp, E. G., Chisholm, D. J., Freund, J., & Boutcher, S. H. (2008). The effects of high-intensity intermittent exercise training on fat loss and fasting insulin levels of young women. *International Journal of Obesity*, 32(4), 684-691.

15. Holliday, A., & Blannin, A. (2017). Very Low Volume Sprint Interval Exercise Suppresses Subjective Appetite, Lowers Acylated Ghrelin, and Elevates GLP-1 in Overweight Individuals: A Pilot Study. *Nutrients*, 9(4), 362.

16. Keating, S. E., Johnson, N. A., Mielke, G. I., & Coombes, J. S. (2017). A systematic review and meta-analysis of interval training versus moderate-intensity continuous training on body adiposity. *Obesity Reviews*, 18(8), 943-964.

17. Jensen MK, Koh-Banerjee P, Franz M, Sampson L, Grønbaek M, Rimm EB. 2006. Whole grains, bran, and germ in relation to homocysteine and markers of glycemic control, lipids, and inflammation 1. *Am. J. Clin. Nutr.* Feb; 83(2):275-83

18. Flight I, Clifton P. 2006. Cereal grains and legumes in the prevention of coronary heart disease and stroke: a review of the literature. *Eur. J. Clin. Nutr.* Oct; 60(10):1145-59

19. Ye E.Q., Chacko S.A., Chou E.L., Kugizaki M., Liu S. 2012. Greater whole-grain intake is associated with lower risk of type 2 diabetes, cardiovascular disease, and weight gain. *J. Nutr.* Jul; 142(7):1304-13.

20. Bray, G. A., & Bouchard, C. (2014). *Handbook of obesity: Clinical applications*. Boca Raton, Florida: CRC Press.

21. Davis, W. J., Wood, D. T., Andrews, R. G., Elkind, L. M., & Davis, W. B. (2008). Concurrent Training Enhances Athletes' Strength, Muscle Endurance, and Other Measures. *Journal of Strength and Conditioning Research*, 22(5), 1487-1502.

22. Davis, W. J., Wood, D. T., Andrews, R. G., Elkind, L. M., & Davis, W. B. (2008). Elimination of Delayed-Onset Muscle Soreness by Pre-resistance Cardioacceleration before Each Set. *Journal of Strength and Conditioning Research*, 22(1), 212-225.

23. Vyas, D., Kadegowda, A. K. G., & Erdman, R. A. (2012). Dietary Conjugated Linoleic Acid and Hepatic Steatosis: Species-Specific Effects on Liver and Adipose Lipid Metabolism and Gene Expression. *Journal of Nutrition and Metabolism*, 2012, 932928.

24. Larsen, T. M., Toubro, S., Gudmundsen, O., & Astrup, A. (2006). Conjugated linoleic acid supplementation for 1 y does not prevent weight or body fat regain. *The American Journal of Clinical Nutrition*, 83(3), 606-612.

25. Villani, R. G., Gannon, J., Self, M., & Rich, P. A. (2000). L-Carnitine Supplementation Combined with Aerobic Training Does Not Promote Weight Loss in Moderately Obese Women. *International Journal of Sport Nutrition and Exercise Metabolism*, 10(2), 199-207.

26. Malaguarnera, M., Cammalleri, L., Gargante, M. P., Vacante, M., Colonna, V., & Motta, M. (2007). L-Carnitine treatment reduces severity of physical and mental fatigue and increases cognitive functions in centenarians: A randomized and controlled clinical trial. *The American Journal of Clinical Nutrition*, 86(6), 1738-1744.

27. Reis, V., Júnior, R., Zajac, A., & Oliveira, D. (2011). Energy Cost of Resistance Exercises: An Update. *Journal of Human Kinetics*, 29A(Special Issue).

28. Schoenfeld, B. J., Ogborn, D., & Krieger, J. W. (2016). Effects of Resistance Training Frequency on Measures of Muscle Hypertrophy: A Systematic Review and Meta-Analysis. *Sports Medicine*, Nov;46(11), 1689-1697.

29. Otsuka, R., Tamakoshi, K., Yatsuya, H., Murata, C., Sekiya, A., Wada, K., & Toyoshima, H. (2006). Eating fast leads to obesity: findings based on self-administered questionnaires among middle-aged Japanese men and women. *Journal of Epidemiology*, 16(3), 117-124.

30. Spiegel, T. A., Wadden, T. A., & Foster, G. D. (1991). Objective measurement of eating rate during behavioral treatment of obesity. *Behavior Therapy*, 22(1), 61-67.

31. Weight management: Lifestyle services for overweight or obese adults. (n.d.). Retrieved January 18, 2018, from https://www.nice.org.uk/guidance/ph53

32. Rshikesan, P. (2016). Yoga Practice for Reducing the Male Obesity and Weight Related Psychological Difficulties-A Randomized Controlled Trial. *Journal of Clinical and Diagnostic Research*.

33. Ross, A., Brooks, A., Touchton-Leonard, K., & Wallen, G. (2016). A Different Weight Loss Experience: A Qualitative Study Exploring the Behavioral, Physical, and Psychosocial Changes Associated with Yoga That Promote Weight Loss. *Evidence-Based Complementary and Alternative Medicine*: eCAM, 2016, 2914745.

34. Barnosky, A. R., Hoddy, K. K., Unterman, I. G., & Varady, K. A. (2014). Intermittent fasting vs daily calorie restriction for type 2 diabetes prevention: A review of human findings. *Translational Research*, 164(4), 302-311.

35. Varady, K. A., Bhutani, S., Church, E. C., & Klempel, M. C. (2009). Short-term modified alternate-day fasting: A novel dietary strategy for weight loss and cardioprotection in obese adults. *The American Journal of Clinical Nutrition*, 90(5), 1138-1143.

36. Johnstone, A. (2014). Fasting for weight loss: An effective strategy or latest dieting trend? *International Journal of Obesity*, 39(5), 727-733.

37. Vispute, S. S., Smith, J. D., Lecheminant, J. D., & Hurley, K. S. (2011). The Effect of Abdominal Exercise on Abdominal Fat. *Journal of Strength and Conditioning Research*, 25(9), 2559-2564.

38. Schoenfeld, B. J., Aragon, A. A., Krieger, J. W., (2015). Effects of meal frequency on weight loss and body composition: A meta-analysis. *Nutrition Reviews*, Volume 73, Issue (2), 1, Pages 69–82

39. Sofer, S., Eliraz, A., Kaplan, S., Voet, H., Fink, G., Kima, T., & Madar, Z. (2011). Greater Weight Loss and Hormonal Changes After 6 Months Diet With Carbohydrates Eaten Mostly at Dinner. *Obesity*, 19(10), 2006-2014.

40. Aragon, A. A., Schoenfeld, B. J., (2013). Nutrient timing revisited: Is there a post-exercise anabolic window?. *Journal of the International Society of Sports Nutrition*, 10 (5).

41. Stewart, T. M., Williamson, D. A., & White, M. A. (2002). Rigid vs. flexible dieting: Association with eating disorder symptoms in nonobese women. *Appetite*, 38(1), 39-44.

42. Meule, A., Westenhöfer, J., & Kübler, A. (2011). Food cravings mediate the relationship between rigid, but not flexible control of eating behavior and dieting success. *Appetite*, 57(3), 582-584.

43. Powers, T. A., Koestner, R., & Gorin, A. A. (2008). Autonomy support from family and friends and weight loss in college women. *Families, Systems, & Health*, 26(4), 404-416.

44. Wing, R. R., & Jeffery, R. W. (1999). Benefits of recruiting participants with friends and increasing social support for weight loss and maintenance. *Journal of Consulting and Clinical Psychology*,67(1), 132-138.

45. Trexler, E. T., Smith-Ryan, A. E., Norton, L.E. (2014). Metabolic adaptation to weight loss: Implications for the athlete. *Journal of the International Society of Sports Nutrition*. Feb 27;11(1), 7

46. Villablanca, P. A., Alegria, J. R., Mookadam, F., Holmes, D. R., Wright, R. S., & Levine, J. A. (2015). Nonexercise Activity Thermogenesis in Obesity Management. *Mayo Clinic Proceedings*, 90(4), 509-519.

47. Trexler, E. T., Smith-Ryan, A. E., Norton, L.E. (2014). Metabolic adaptation to weight loss: implications for the athlete. *Journal of the International Society of Sports Nutrition*. Feb 27;11(1):7

48. Doucet, E., Imbeault, P., St-Pierre, S., Alméras, N., Mauriège, P., Després, J., & Tremblay, A. (2003). Greater than predicted decrease in energy expenditure during exercise after body weight loss in obese men. *Clinical Science*,105(1), 89-95.

49. Aragon, A. A., Schoenfeld, B. J., (2013). Nutrient timing revisited: Is there a post-exercise anabolic window? *Journal of the International Society of Sports Nutrition*, 10(5).

50. Trommelen, J., van Loon, L. J. C. (2016). Pre-Sleep Protein Ingestion to Improve the Skeletal Muscle Adaptive Response to Exercise Training. *Nutrients*, 8(12), 763.

51. Wang, H., Wen, Y., Du, Y., Yan, X., Guo, H., Rycroft, J. A., & Mela, D. J.

(2009). Effects of Catechin Enriched Green Tea on Body Composition. *Obesity*, 18(4), 773-779.

52. Jurgens, T. M., Whelan, A. M., Kirk, S., & Foy, E. (2010). Green tea for weight loss and weight maintenance in overweight or obese adults. *Cochrane Database of Systematic Reviews*.

53. Calatayud, J., Borreani, S., Colado, J. C., Martín, F. F., Rogers, M. E., Behm, D. G., & Andersen, L. L. (2014). Muscle Activation during Push-Ups with Different Suspension Training Systems. *Journal of Sports Science & Medicine*, 13(3), 502-510.

54. Skorka-Brown, J., Andrade, J., May, J. (2014). Playing Tetris® reduces the strength, frequency and vividness of naturally occurring cravings. *Appetite*. 76:161–5.

55. Andrade, J., Pears, S., May, J., & Kavanagh, D. J. (2012). Use of a clay modeling task to reduce chocolate craving. *Appetite*, 58(3), 955-963.

56. FoodT brain training app (n.d.). Retrieved November 22, 2017, from https://www.exeter.ac.uk/foodt

57. Anderson, J. W., Baird, P., Davis, R. H., Ferreri, S., Knudtson, M., Koraym, A., Waters, V., Williams, C. L. (2009). Health benefits of dietary fiber. *Nutrition Reviews*, 67, 188-205.

58. Clark, M. J., & Slavin, J. L. (2013). The effect of fiber on satiety and food intake: A systematic review. *Journal of the American College of Nutrition*, 32(3), 200-211.

59. How to get more fibre into your diet – Live Well. (n.d.). Retrieved April 18, 2018, from https://www.nhs.uk/chq/pages/1141.aspx?categoryid=51

60. Carey, D. G. (2009). Quantifying differences in the 'fat burning' zone and the aerobic zone: implications for training. *J. Strength Cond. Res.* Oct; 23(7):2090-95.

61. Retrieved from www.pnas.org/content/arly/2009/11/06/0908789106

62. Retrieved from www.ncbi.nlm.nih.gov/pmc/articles/PMC4013785/

63. What is CrossFit? (n.d.). Retrieved November 22, 2017, from https://www.crossfit.com/what-is-crossfit

64. Smith, M. M., Sommer, A. J., Starkoff, B. E., Devor, S. T. (2013). CrossFit-based high-intensity power training improves maximal aerobic fitness and body composition. *Journal*

of Strength and Conditioning Research, 27, 3159-3172

65. Meyer, J., Morrison, J., Zuniga, J. (2017) The Benefits and Risks of CrossFit: A Systematic Review. *Workplace Health Saf.* Dec; 65(12):612-618.

66. Aune, D., Giovannucci, E., Boffetta, P., et al (2017). Fruit and vegetable intake and the risk of cardiovascular disease, total cancer and all-cause mortality – a systematic review and dose-response meta-analysis of prospective studies. *International Journal of Epidemiology*; 46:1029-56

67. Swinburn, B., Eggar, G., & Raza., F. (1999). Dissecting obesogenic environments; the development and application of a framework for identifying and prioritizing environmental interventions for obesity. *Preventive Medicine*, 29(6), 563-570

68. Wansink, B., Hanks, A. S., & Kaipainen, K. (2016). Slim by Design. *Health Education & Behavior*, 43(5), 552-558.

69. Block, J. P., Condon, S. K., Kleinman, K., et al. (2013). Consumers' estimation of calorie content at fast food restaurants: Cross sectional observational study. *British Medical Journal*, 346, f2907.

70. Buhl, K. M., Gallagher, D., Hoy, K., Matthews, D. E., Heymsfield. S. (1995). Unexplained disturbance in body weight regulation: diagnostic outcome assessed by doubly labeled water and body composition analyses in obese patients reporting low energy intakes. *Journal of the American Dietetic Association* 95, 1393-1400.

71. Champagne, C. M., Bray, G.A., Kurtz, A.A., et al. (2002). Energy intake and energy expenditure: a controlled study comparing dietitians and non-dietitians. *J. Am. Diet. Assoc.* 102:1428-1432

72. Holden, S. S., Zlatevska, N., & Dubelaar, C. (2016). Whether Smaller Plates Reduce Consumption Depends on Who's Serving and Who's Looking: A Meta-Analysis. *Journal of the Association for Consumer Research*, 1(1), 134-146.

73. File:Delboeuf illusion.svg. (n.d.). Retrieved April 18, 2018, from https://commons.wikimedia.org/wiki/File:Delboeuf_illusion.svg

74. Hobson, R. (2017, January). Yes, you CAN eat carbs! Expert reveals the 5

best recipes to keep you slim and full of energy – and stop you getting 'hangry' *The Daily Mail*. Retrieved November 30, 2017, from http://www.dailymail.co.uk/health/article-4160448/Expert-reveals-eat-carbs-stay-slim.html

75. Thomson, K. (2016, July). Cut carbs, quit sugar, feel fabulous: It's a food revolution that'll make you slimmer and happier - and it's blissfully simple. *The Daily Mail*. Retrieved November 30, 2017, from http://www.dailymail.co.uk/femail/food/article-3672595/Cut-carbs-quit-sugar-feel-fabulous-s-food-revolution-ll-make-slimmer-happier-s-blissfully-simple.html

76. Cooper, B. E. J., Lee, W. E., Goldacre, B. M., Sanders, T. A. (2012) The quality of the evidence for dietary advice given in UK national newspapers. *Public Understanding of Science*, 21:664-73

77. Wansink, B., van Kleef, E. (2014). Dinner rituals that correlate with child and adult BMI. *Obesity* (Silver Spring). 22(5):E91-E95

78. Bowman, S. A. (2006). Television-viewing characteristics of adults: correlations to eating practices and overweight and health status. *Preventing Chronic Disease*, 3(2):A38.

79. Wansink, B. (2004). Environmental factors that increase the food intake and consumption volume of unknowing consumers. *Annual Review of Nutrition*, 24:455-479.

80. Bodenlos, J., Wormuth, B. (2013). Watching a food-related television show and caloric intake. A laboratory study. *Appetite*, 61, 8-12

81. Mathur, U., Stevenson, R. J. (2015). Television and eating: repetition enhances food intake. *Frontiers in Psychology*, 6, 1657.

82. Harris J., Bargh J., Brownell K. (2009). Priming effects of television food advertising on eating behavior. *Health Psychol.* 28, 404–413.

83. Weight management: Lifestyle services for overweight or obese adults. (n.d.). Retrieved January 18, 2018, from https://www.nice.org.uk/guidance/ph53

84. Jones, A. M., Doust, J. H. (1996). A 1% treadmill grade most accurately reflects the energetic cost of outdoor running. *Journal of Sports Sciences*, 14(4), 321-327.

85. Maas, J. (2006). Green space, urbanity, and health: How strong is the relation? *Journal of Epidemiology & Community Health*, 60(7), 587-592.

86. Barton, J., Pretty, J. (2010). What is the best dose of nature and green exercise for improving mental health? A multi-study analysis. *Environmental Science and Technology*, 44, 10, 3947-3955.

87. Holick, M. F. (2007). Vitamin D deficiency. *The New England Journal of Medicine*. 357:266-81.

88. Kerr, D.C., et al. (2015). Associations between vitamin D levels and depressive symptoms in healthy young adult women. *Psychiatry Research*, 227, 1, 46-51.

89. Armstrong, R. B. (1984). Mechanisms of exercise-induced delayed onset muscular soreness. *Medicine & Science in Sports Exercise*, 16:529–538

90. Duncan, G. E. (2005). Prescribing Exercise at Varied Levels of Intensity and Frequency. *Archives of Internal Medicine*, 165(20), 2362.

91. Dishman, R. K. (2010). Psychological factors and physical activity level. *In Physical Activity and Obesity* (pp. 89-93). IL: Human Kinetics.

92. Tribole E., Resch, E. (2003). *Intuitive eating: a revolutionary program that works*. St. Martin's Griffin New York.

93. Van Dyke, N., Drinkwater, E.J., (2014). Relationships between intuitive eating and health indicators: literature review. *Public health nutrition*. 17(8):1757–1766

94. Tracy, B. (2007). *Eat that Frog!: 21 Great Ways to Stop Procrastinating and Get More Done in Less Time* (2nd ed.). Berrett-Koehler Publishers.

95. Alizadeh, Z., Mostafaee, M., Mazaheri, R., & Younespour, S. (2015). Acute Effect of Morning and Afternoon Aerobic Exercise on Appetite of Overweight Women. *Asian Journal of Sports Medicine*,6(2). doi: 10.5812/asjsm.6(2)20156.24222

96. Seo, D. Y., Lee, S., Kim, N., Ko, K. S., Rhee, B. D., Park, B. J., & Han, J. (2013). Morning and evening exercise. *Integrative Medicine Research*, 2(4), 139-144.

97. Schoenfeld, B., Aragon, A., Wilborn, C. D., Krieger, J. W., & Sonmez, G. T. (2014). Body composition changes associated with fasted versus non-fasted aerobic exercise. *Journal of the International Society of Sports Nutrition*, 11(1), 54.

98. Calaprice, A. (2010). *The Ultimate Quotable Einstein*. Princeton: Princeton University Press

99. Peterson, M. D., Pistilli, E., Haff, G. G., Hoffman, E. P., & Gordon, P. M. (2011). Progression of volume load and muscular adaptation during resistance exercise. *European Journal of Applied Physiology*, 111(6), 1063-1071.

100. Rhodes, R. E., & Pfaeffli, L. A. (2010). Mediators of physical activity behaviour change among adult non-clinical populations: A review update. *International Journal of Behavioral Nutrition and Physical Activity*, 7(1), 37.

101. Mozaffarian, D., Hao, T., Rimm, E. B., Willett, W. C., & Hu, F. B. (2011). Changes in Diet and Lifestyle and Long-Term Weight Gain in Women and Men. *New England Journal of Medicine*, 364(25), 2392-2404.

102. Knutson, K. L., & Cauter, E. V. (2008). Associations between Sleep Loss and Increased Risk of Obesity and Diabetes. *Annals of the New York Academy of Sciences*, 1129(1), 287-304.

103. Sharma, S., Kavuru, M. (2010). Sleep and Metabolism: An Overview. *International Journal of Endocrinology*, 2010, 270832.

104. Nedeltcheva, A. V., Kilkus, J. M., Imperial, J., Kasza, K., Schoeller, D. A., & Penev, P. D. (2008). Sleep curtailment is accompanied by increased intake of calories from snacks. *The American Journal of Clinical Nutrition*,89(1), 126-133.

105. Halson, S. L. (2014). Sleep in Elite Athletes and Nutritional Interventions to Enhance Sleep. *Sports Medicine* (Auckland, NZ), 44(Suppl 1), 13-23.

106. Chang, A., Aeschbach, D., Duffy, J. F., & Czeisler, C. A. (2014). Evening use of light-emitting eReaders negatively affects sleep, circadian timing, and next-morning alertness. *Proceedings of the National Academy of Sciences*, 112(4), 1232-1237.

107. Lemon, P. W. (2000). Beyond the Zone: Protein Needs of Active Individuals. *Journal of the American College of Nutrition*, 19(Sup5).

108. Schoenfeld, B. J., Ratamess, N. A., Peterson, M. D., Contreras, B., Sonmez, G. T., & Alvar, B. A. (2014). Effects of Different Volume-Equated Resistance Training Loading Strategies on Muscular

Adaptations in Well-Trained Men. *Journal of Strength and Conditioning Research*, 28(10), 2909-2918.

109. Rawson, E. S., & Volek, J. S. (2003). Effects of Creatine Supplementation and Resistance Training on Muscle Strength and Weightlifting Performance. *The Journal of Strength and Conditioning Research*, 17(4), 822.

110. Branch, J. D. (2003). Effect of creatine supplementation on body composition and performance: a meta-analysis. *International Journal of Sport Nutrition and Exercise Metabolism*. Jun; 13(2):198-226.

111. Adams, S. (2014). *How to fail at almost everything and still win big: Kind of the story of my life*. New York, NY: Portfolio/Penguin

112. Guise, S., 2016. *Mini Habits for Weight Loss: Stop Dieting*. 2nd ed. Selective Entertainment LLC

113. Ducrot, P., Méjean, C., Aroumougame, V., Ibanez, G., Allès, B., Kesse-Guyot, E., & Péneau, S. (2017). Meal planning is associated with food variety, diet quality and body weight status in a large sample of French adults. *The International Journal of Behavioral Nutrition and Physical Activity*, 14, 12.

114. The Weider Principles. (n.d.). Retrieved December 12, 2017, from https://www.muscleandfitness.com/workouts/workout-tips/weider-principles

115. Metz, E. (2015, March 28). Why Singapore banned chewing gum. Retrieved January 18, 2018, from http://www.bbc.co.uk/news/magazine-32090420

116. Park, E., Edirisinghe, I., Inui, T., Kergoat, S., Kelley, M., & Burton-Freeman, B. (2016). Short-term effects of chewing gum on satiety and afternoon snack intake in healthy weight and obese women. *Physiology & Behavior*, 159, 64-71.

117. Xu, J., Xiao, X., Li, Y., Zheng, J., Li, W., Zhang, Q., & Wang, Z. (2015). The effect of gum chewing on blood GLP-1 concentration in fasted, healthy, non-obese men. *Endocrine*, 50(1), 93-98.

118. Bauditz, J., Norman, K., Biering, H., Lochs, H., & Pirlich, M. (2008). Severe weight loss caused by chewing gum. *British Medical Journal*, 336(7635), 96-97.

119. Byrne, N. M., Sainsbury, A., King, N. A., Hills, A. P., & Wood, R. E. (2017). Intermittent energy restriction improves weight loss efficiency in obese men: The MATADOR study. *International Journal of Obesity*, 42(2), 129-138.

120. Tal, A., & Wansink, B. (2013). Fattening Fasting: Hungry Grocery Shoppers Buy More Calories, Not More Food. *JAMA Internal Medicine*, 173(12), 1146.

121. Tal, A., & Wansink, B. (2015). An Apple a Day Brings More Apples Your Way: Healthy Samples Prime Healthier Choices. *Psychology & Marketing*, 32(5), 575-584.

122. Wansink, B., Soman, D., & Herbst, K. C. (2017). Larger partitions lead to larger sales: Divided grocery carts alter purchase norms and increase sales. *Journal of Business Research*, 75, 202-209.

123. Gorin, A. A., Raynor, H. A., Niemeier, H. M., & Wing, R. R. (2007). Home grocery delivery improves the household food environments of behavioral weight loss participants: Results of an 8-week pilot study. *The International Journal of Behavioral Nutrition and Physical Activity*, 4, 58.

124. Lee, B. A., Oh, D. J. (2015). Effect of regular swimming exercise on the physical composition, strength, and blood lipid of middle-aged women. *Journal of Exercise Rehabilitation*, 11(5), 266-271.

125. Cox, K. L., Burke, V., Beilin, L. J., Puddey, I.B. (2010). A comparison of the effects of swimming and walking on body weight, fat distribution, lipids, glucose, and insulin in older women – the Sedentary Women Exercise Adherence Trial 2. *Metabolism*. Nov;59(11):1562-73.

126. Segura, R., Javierre, C., Lizarraga, M. A., & Ros, E. (2006). Other relevant components of nuts: Phytosterols, folate and minerals. *British Journal of Nutrition*, 96(S2).

127. Alper, C., & Mattes, R. (2002). Effects of chronic peanut consumption on energy balance and hedonics. *International Journal of Obesity*, 26(8), 1129-1137.

128. Scrafford, C. G., Tran, N. L., Barraj, L. M., & Mink, P. J. (2010). Egg consumption and CHD and stroke mortality: A prospective study of US adults. *Public Health Nutrition*,14(02), 261-270. doi:10.1017/

s1368980010001874

129. Blesso, C. N., Andersen, C. J., Barona, J., Volek, J. S., & Fernandez, M. L. (2013). Whole egg consumption improves lipoprotein profiles and insulin sensitivity to a greater extent than yolk-free egg substitute in individuals with metabolic syndrome. *Metabolism*, 62(3), 400-410.

130. Schoenfeld, B. J., Aragon, A. A., Wilborn, C. D., Krieger, J. W., & Sonmez, G. T. (2014). Body composition changes associated with fasted versus non-fasted aerobic exercise. *Journal of the International Society of Sports Nutrition*, 11, 54.

131. Vliet, S. V., Burd, N. A., & Loon, L. J. (2015). The Skeletal Muscle Anabolic Response to Plant- versus Animal-Based Protein Consumption. *The Journal of Nutrition*, 145(9), 1981-1991.

132. Biston, P., Cauter, E. V., Ofek, G., Linkowski, P., Polonsky, K. S., & Degaute, J. (1996). Diurnal Variations in Cardiovascular Function and Glucose Regulation in Normotensive Humans. *Hypertension*, 28(5), 863-871.

133. Davy, B. M., Dennis, E. A., Dengo, A. L., Wilson, K. L., & Davy, K. P. (2008). Water Consumption Reduces Energy Intake at a Breakfast Meal in Obese Older Adults. *Journal of the American Dietetic Association*, 108(7), 1236-1239.

134. Lappalainen, R., Mennen, L., van Weert, L., Mykkanen, H. (1993) Drinking water with a meal: A simple method of coping with feelings of hunger, satiety and desire to eat. *European Journal of Clinical Nutrition*, 47:815-819

135. Popkin, B. M., Barclay, D. V., & Nielsen, S. J. (2005). Water and Food Consumption Patterns of U.S. Adults from 1999 to 2001. *Obesity Research*, 13(12), 2146-2152.

136. Stookey, J. D., Constant, F., Popkin, B. M., & Gardner, C. D. (2008). Drinking Water Is Associated With Weight Loss in Overweight Dieting Women Independent of Diet and Activity. *Obesity*, 16(11), 2481-2488.

137. Muckelbauer, R., Libuda, L., Clausen, K., Toschke, A. M., Reinehr, T., & Kersting, M. (2012). Promotion and Provision of Drinking Water in Schools for Overweight Prevention. *Nutrition Today*, 47.

138. Probably the Toughest Event on The Planet. (n.d.). Retrieved March 7, 2018, from https://toughmudder.co.uk/events/what-is-tough-mudder

139. Hollis, J. F., Gullion, C. M., Stevens, V. J., Brantley, P. J., Appel, L. J., Ard, J. D., & Svetkey, L. P. (2008). Weight Loss During the Intensive Intervention Phase of the Weight-Loss Maintenance Trial. *American Journal of Preventive Medicine*, 35(2), 118-126.

140. Brits lose count of their calories: Over a third of Brits don't know how many calories they consume on a typical day. (n.d.). Retrieved April 12, 2018, from http://www.mintel.com/press-centre/food-and-drink/brits-lose-count-of-their-calories-over-a-third-of-brits-dont-know-how-many-calories-they-consume-on-a-typical-day

141. Block, J. P., Condon, S. K., Kleinman, K., Mullen, J., Linakis, S., Rifas-Shiman, S., & Gillman, M. W. (2013). Consumers' estimation of calorie content at fast food restaurants: Cross sectional observational study. *British Medical Journal*, 346(May 23;346).

142. Burke, L. E., Wang, J., & Sevick, M. A. (2011). Self-Monitoring in Weight Loss: A Systematic Review of the Literature. *Journal of the American Dietetic Association*, 111(1), 92-102.

143. Sharma, H. (2015). Meditation: Process and effects. *Ayu*, 36(3), 233-237.

144. Kaufman, K.A., Glass, C.R., Arnkoff, D.B. (2009). Evaluation of Mindful Sport Performance Enhancement (MSPE). A New Approach to Promote Flow in Athletes. *Journal of Clinical Sport Psychology*, 3/4:334–356.

145. Spadaro, K. C., Davis, K. K., Sereika, S. M., Gibbs, B. B., Jakicic, J. M., & Cohen, S. M. (2017). Effect of mindfulness meditation on short-term weight loss and eating behaviors in overweight and obese adults: A randomized controlled trial. *Journal of Complementary and Integrative Medicine*, 0(0).

146. Frappier, J., Toupin, I., Levy, J. J., Aubertin-Leheudre, M., Karelis, A. D. (2013). Energy Expenditure during Sexual Activity in Young Healthy Couples. *Plos One*, 8(10), e79342

147. Hambach, A., Evers, S., Summ, O., Husstedt, I. W., Frese, A. (2013). The impact of sexual activity on idiopathic headaches: an observational study. *Cephalalgia*. Apr;33(6):384-9.

148. Wright, H., Jenks, R. A. (2016). Sex on the brain! Associations between sexual activity and cognitive function in older age. *Age Ageing*. 2016 Mar;45(2):313-7.

149. Gardner, C. D., Trepanowski, J. F., Gobbo, L. C., Hauser, M. E., Rigdon, J., Ioannidis, J. P., & King, A. C. (2018). Effect of Low-Fat vs Low-Carbohydrate Diet on 12-Month Weight Loss in Overweight Adults and the Association With Genotype Pattern or Insulin Secretion. *Jama*, 319(7), 667.

150. Hall, K. D., Chen, K. Y., Guo, J., Lam, Y. Y., Leibel, R. L., Mayer, L. E., & Ravussin, E. (2016). Energy expenditure and body composition changes after an isocaloric ketogenic diet in overweight and obese men. *The American Journal of Clinical Nutrition*, 104(2), 324-333.

151. Fat: The facts – Live Well. (n.d.). Retrieved April 3, 2018, from https://www.nhs.uk/Livewell/Goodfood/Pages/Fat.aspx

152. Gallo-Reynoso, J., & Ortiz, C. L. (2010). Feral cats steal milk from northern Elephant Seals. *Therya*,1(3), 207-212.

153. Thorning, T. K., Raben, A., Tholstrup, T., Soedamah-Muthu, S. S., Givens, I., & Astrup, A. (2016). Milk and dairy products: good or bad for human health? An assessment of the totality of scientific evidence. *Food & Nutrition Research*, 60.

154. Stonehouse, W., Wycherley, T., Luscombe-Marsh, N., Taylor, P., Brinkworth, G., & Riley, M. (2016). Dairy Intake Enhances Body Weight and Composition Changes during Energy Restriction in 18–50-Year-Old Adults—A Meta-Analysis of Randomized Controlled Trials. *Nutrients*, 8(7), 394.

155. Schwingshackl, L., Hoffmann, G., Schwedhelm, C., Kalle-Uhlmann, T., Missbach, B., Knüppel, S., & Boeing, H. (2016). Consumption of Dairy Products in Relation to Changes in Anthropometric Variables in Adult Populations: A Systematic Review and Meta-Analysis of Cohort Studies. *Plos One*, 11(6).

156. Smith, A. E., Fukuda, D. H., Kendall, K. L., & Stout, J. R. (2010). The effects of a pre-workout supplement containing caffeine, creatine, and amino acids during three weeks of high-intensity exercise on aerobic and anaerobic performance. *Journal of the International Society of Sports Nutrition*, 7, 10.

157. International Association of Athletics Federation. *Nutrition for Athletics: A Practical Guide to Eating for Health and Performance.* Monaco: IAAF; 2016

158. Harpaz, E., Tamir, S., Weinstein, A., & Weinstein, Y. (2017). The effect of caffeine on energy balance. *Journal of Basic and Clinical Physiology and Pharmacology*, 28(1), 1-10.

159. Pareja-Blanco, F., Rodríguez-Rosell, D., Sánchez-Medina, L., Sanchis-Moysi, J., Dorado, C., Mora-Custodio, R., González-Badillo, J. J. (2016). Effects of velocity loss during resistance training on athletic performance, strength gains and muscle adaptations. *Scandinavian Journal of Medicine & Science in Sports*, 27(7), 724-735.

160. Weakley, J. J. S., Till, K., Read, D. B., Roe, G. A. B., Darrall-Jones, J., Phibbs, P. J., & Jones, B. (2017). The effects of traditional, superset, and tri-set resistance training structures on perceived intensity and physiological responses. *European Journal of Applied Physiology*, 117(9), 1877-1889.

161. Kelleher, A. R., Hackney, K. J., Fairchild, T. J., Keslacy, S., & Ploutz-Snyder, L. L. (2010). The Metabolic Costs of Reciprocal Supersets vs. Traditional Resistance Exercise in Young Recreationally Active Adults. *Journal of Strength and Conditioning Research*, 24(4), 1043-1051.

162. Maia, M. F., Willardson, J. M., Paz, G. A., & Miranda, H. (2014). Effects of Different Rest Intervals Between Antagonist Paired Sets on Repetition Performance and Muscle Activation. *Journal of Strength and Conditioning Research*, 28(9), 2529-2535.

163. Magnuson, B. A., Burdock, G. A., Doull, J., Kroes, R. M., Marsh, G. M., Pariza, M. W., & Williams, G. M. (2007). Aspartame: A safety evaluation based on current use levels, regulations, and toxicological and epidemiological studies. *Critical Reviews in Toxicology*, 37(8), 629-727

164. Bouzari, A., Holstege, D., & Barrett, D. M. (2015). Mineral, Fiber, and Total Phenolic Retention in Eight Fruits and Vegetables: A Comparison of Refrigerated and Frozen Storage. *Journal of Agricultural and Food Chemistry*, 63(3), 951-956.

165. Shephard, R. (2012). 2011 Compendium of Physical Activities: A Second Update of Codes and MET Values. *Yearbook of Sports Medicine*, 2012, 126-127.

166. Friedenreich, C. M. (2011) Physical activity and breast cancer: review of the epidemiologic evidence and biologic mechanisms. *Recent Results in Cancer Research.* 188:125-39

167. Healy, G. N., Winkler, E. A., Owen, N., Anuradha, S., & Dunstan, D. W. (2015). Replacing sitting time with standing or stepping: Associations with cardio-metabolic risk biomarkers. *European Heart Journal*, 36(39), 2643-2649.

168. Office workers spend too much time at their desks, experts say. (2012, January 15). Retrieved April 8, 2017, from http://www.sciencedaily.com/releases/2012/01/120113210203.htm

169. Eating Soup Will Help Cut Calories At Meals. (2007, May 02). Retrieved April 6, 2018, from http://www.sciencedaily.com/releases/2007/05/070501142326.htm

170. Alhassan, S., Kim, S., Bersamin, A., King, A., & Gardner, C. (2008). Dietary adherence and weight loss success among overweight women: Results from the A to Z weight loss study. *International Journal of Obesity* (2005), 32(6), 985-991.

171. Zepeda, L., & Deal, D. (2008). Think before you eat: Photographic food diaries as intervention tools to change dietary decision making and attitudes. *International Journal of Consumer Studies*, 32(6), 692-698.

172. Coary, S., & Poor, M. (2016). How consumer-generated images shape important consumption outcomes in the food domain. *Journal of Consumer Marketing*, 33(1), 1-8.

173. Evans, E. M., Mojtahedi, M. C., Thorpe, M. P., Valentine, R. J., Kris-Etherton, P. M., & Layman, D. K. (2012). Effects of protein intake and gender on body composition changes: a randomized clinical weight loss trial. *Nutrition & Metabolism*, 9, 55.

174. Halvorsen, B. L., Blomhoff, R. (2011). Determination of lipid oxidation products in vegetable oils and marine omega-3 supplements. *Food & Nutrition Research*, 55, 2.

175. Tsuji, H., Kasai, M., Takeuchi, H., Nakamura, M., Okazaki, M., & Kondo, K. (2001). Dietary Medium-Chain Triacylglycerols Suppress Accumulation of Body Fat in a Double-Blind, Controlled Trial in Healthy Men and Women. *The Journal of Nutrition*, 131(11), 2853-2859.

176. Valente, F. X., Cândido, F. G., Lopes, L. L., Dias, D. M., Carvalho, S. D., Pereira, P. F., & Bressan, J. (2017). Effects of coconut oil consumption on energy metabolism, cardiometabolic risk markers, and appetitive responses in women with excess body fat. *European Journal of Nutrition*, 1(11).

177. Smith-Spangler, C., Brandeau, M. L., Olkin, I., & Bravata, D. M. (2013). Are Organic Foods Safer or Healthier? *Annals of Internal Medicine*, 158(4), 297.

178. Examine.com. (2018, March 11). Fish Oil - Scientific Review on Usage, Dosage, Side Effects. Retrieved April 10, 2018, from https://examine.com/supplements/fish-oil

179. Simopoulos, A. P. (2008). The Importance of the Omega-6/Omega-3 Fatty Acid Ratio in Cardiovascular Disease and Other Chronic Diseases. *Experimental Biology and Medicine*, 233(6), 674-688.

180. Martins, J. G. (2009). EPA but not DHA appears to be responsible for the efficacy of Omega-3 LC-PUFA supplementation in depression: Evidence from an updated meta-analysis of randomized controlled trials. *Journal of the American College of Nutrition*, 28(5), 525-542.

181. Giuseppe, D. D., Wallin, A., Bottai, M., Askling, J., & Wolk, A. (2013). Long-term intake of dietary long-chain n-3 polyunsaturated fatty acids and risk of rheumatoid arthritis: A prospective cohort study of women. *Annals of the Rheumatic Diseases*, 73(11), 1949-1953.

182. Is oily fish a superfood? – Live Well. (n.d.). Retrieved April 10, 2018, from https://www.nhs.uk/livewell/superfoods/pages/is-oily-fish-a-superfood.aspx

183. Scientific Opinion on the Tolerable Upper Intake Level of eicosapentaenoic acid (EPA), docosahexaenoic acid (DHA) and docosapentaenoic acid (DPA). (2012). *EFSA Journal*, 10(7).

184. Manocchia, P., Spierer, D. K., Lufkin, A. K., Minichiello, J., Castro, J. (2013). Transference of kettlebell training to strength, power, and endurance. *Journal of Strength and Conditioning Research*, Feb;27(2):477-84

185. What is a Kettlebell? (n.d.). Retrieved November 18, 2017, from https://www.kettlebellsusa.com/what-is-a-kettlebell

186. Falatic, J. A., Plato, P. A., Holder, C., Finch, D., Han, K., & Cisar, C. J. (2015). Effects of Kettlebell Training on Aerobic Capacity. *Journal of Strength and Conditioning Research*, 29(7), 1943-1947.

187. Oja, P., Titze, S., Bauman, A., Geus, B. D., Krenn, P., Reger-Nash, B., & Kohlberger, T. (2011). Health benefits of cycling: A systematic review. *Scandinavian Journal of Medicine & Science in Sports*, 21(4), 496-509.

188. Physical Activity and Public Health: Updated Recommendation for Adults from the American College of Sports Medicine and the American Heart Association. (2007). *Circulation*, 116(9), 1081-1093.

189. Speakman, J. R., & Selman, C. (2003). Physical activity and resting metabolic rate. *Proceedings of the Nutrition Society*, 62(3), 621-634.

190. Broom, D. R., Batterham, R. L., King, J. A., & Stensel, D. J. (2009). Influence of resistance and aerobic exercise on hunger, circulating levels of acylated ghrelin, and peptide YY in healthy males. *American Journal of Physiology-Regulatory, Integrative and Comparative Physiology*, 296(1), 29-35.

191. Kalm, L. M., & Semba, R. D. (2005). They Starved So That Others Be Better Fed: Remembering Ancel Keys and the Minnesota Experiment. *The Journal of Nutrition*, 135(6), 1347-1352.

192. Bizzaro, N., Tozzoli, R., Villalta, D., Fabris, M., & Tonutti, E. (2010). Cutting-Edge Issues in Coeliac Disease and in Gluten Intolerance. *Clinical Reviews in Allergy & Immunology*, 42(3), 279-287.

193. Isaac, A. R. (1992). Mental Practice – Does It Work in the Field? *The Sport Psychologist*, 6(2), 192-198.

194. Knäuper, B., Mccollam, A., Rosen-Brown, A., Lacaille, J., Kelso, E., & Roseman, M. (2011). Fruitful plans: Adding targeted mental imagery to implementation intentions increases fruit consumption. *Psychology & Health*, 26(5), 601-617.

INDEX

ACKNOWLEDGEMENTS

Firstly I'd like to thank my amazing wife Becky for her support and for enduring me prattling on about weight-loss habits for months on end. My parents and close friends also need a mention for their enthusiasm and interest in the project, too.

Thanks to Cathryn, my agent – the legend who understood why this book had to be written – and Céline, my editor, for sharing that vision and for bringing this book to life. Without you two none of this would have been possible and you will always have my sincerest gratitude.

My friend – Ian – suggested I write a book the very first time we met. Sorry it took me so long to action your words, Ian, but I am glad that I did and thanks for your help with all author-y stuff.

And finally, thanks to many of the gurus and charlatans for spouting their confusing nonsense promoting FAD diets and pseudoscience. If it wasn't for their BS then I would not have had the opportunity to set the record straight and write a book that counters their claims and actually presents the facts on weight loss.

Publishing Director Sarah Lavelle
Commissioning Editor Céline Hughes
Editorial Assistant Harriet Webster
Designer Nicola Ellis
Photographer Jack Lawson
Author's Stylist Jolanda Coetzer
Production Director Vincent Smith
Production Controller Tom Moore

The publisher would like to thank Origin Fitness for the loan of equipment for the photoshoot.

Medical disclaimer: The content of this book is for your general information and use only. Your use of any information is entirely at your own risk, for which we shall not be liable. It shall be your own responsibility to ensure that information in this book meets your specific requirements. Before taking part in any form of exercise, change of diet or consumption of a nutritional supplement you should always consult your doctor.

Published in 2019 by Quadrille,
an imprint of Hardie Grant Publishing

Quadrille
52–54 Southwark Street
London SE1 1UN
quadrille.com

Cataloguing in Publication Data: a catalogue record for this book is available from the British Library.

Text © Scott Baptie 2019
Photography © Jack Lawson 2019
Design © Quadrille 2019

ISBN 978 1 78713 350 1

Printed in China